Belly Dancing Basics

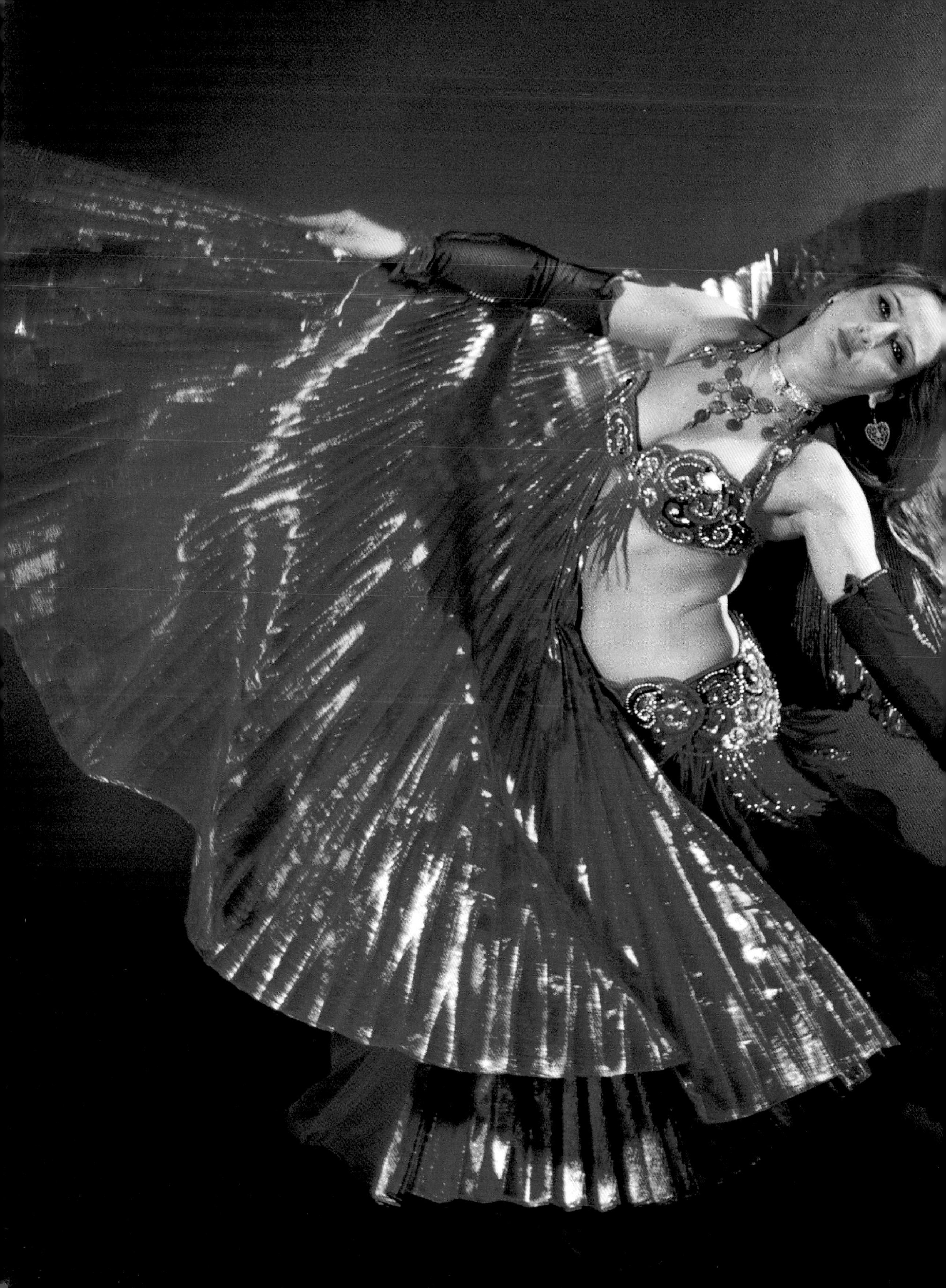

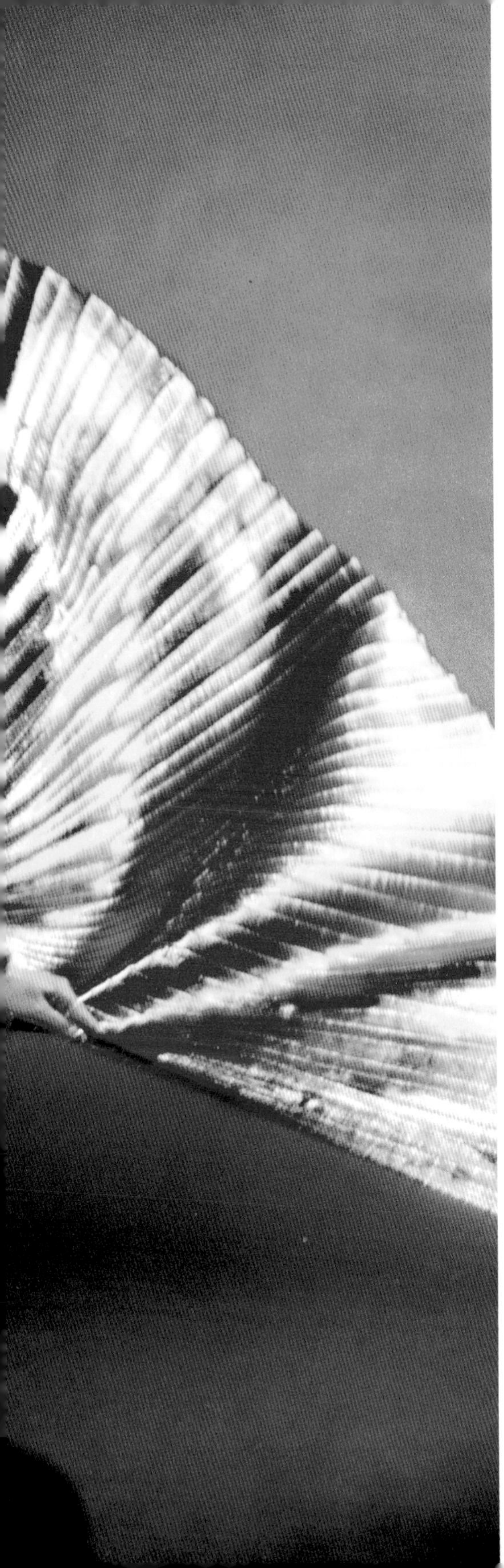

Belly Dancing Basics

Laura A. Cooper

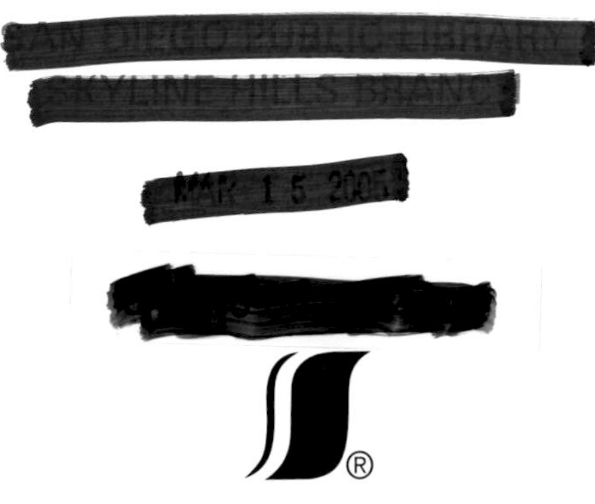

Sterling Publishing Co., Inc.
New York

A GAIA ORIGINAL
Books from Gaia celebrate the vision of Gaia, the self-sustaining living Earth, and seek to help its readers live in greater personal and planetary harmony.

Editor	Jinny Johnson
Designer	Sara Mathews
Photography	Sarah Skinner
Production	Jim Pope
Direction	Joss Pearson, Patrick Nugent

DEDICATION
FOR KIMBERLY

Library of Congress Cataloging-in-Publication Data is Available

10 9 8 7 6 5 4 3 2 1

Published in 2004 by Sterling Publishing Co., Inc.
387 Park Avenue South, New York, N.Y. 10016

Originally published in the United Kingdom in 2004 by
Gaia Books Limited, 66 Charlotte Street, London W1T 4QE

Distributed in Canada by Sterling Publishing
c/o Canadian Manda Group, One Atlantic Avenue, Suite 105
Toronto, Ontario, Canada M6K 3E7

Printed in Singapore by Imago

Sterling ISBN 1-4027-1078-X

CAUTION
Belly dance is generally a safe form of exercise for healthy women. If, however, you have back problems or you are in any doubt about your medical condition, check with your doctor before starting belly dance. Most women can also continue belly dancing while pregnant but, again, check with your doctor to make sure.

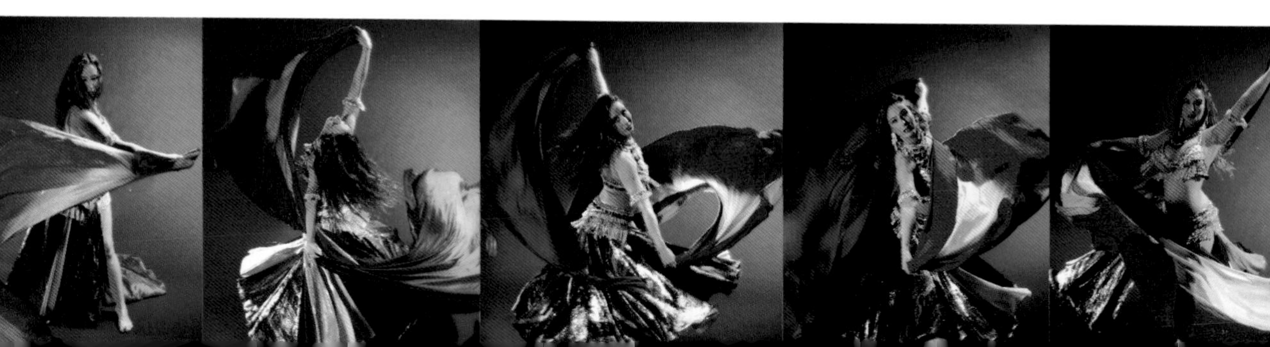

Contents

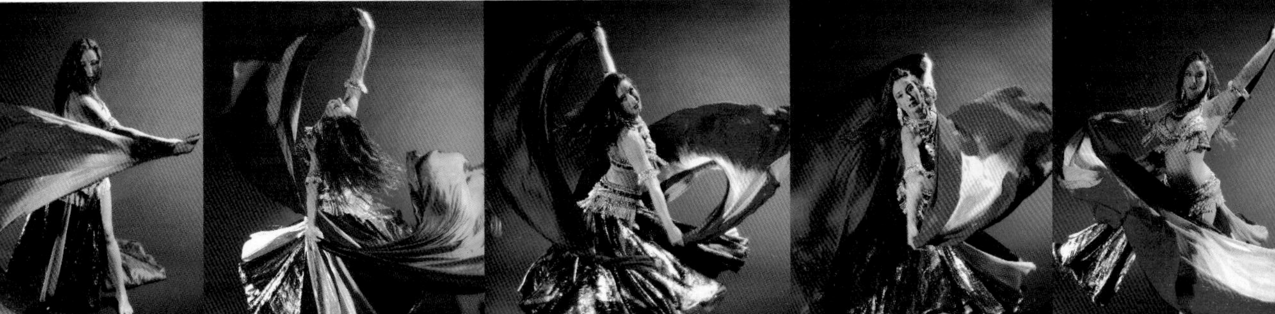

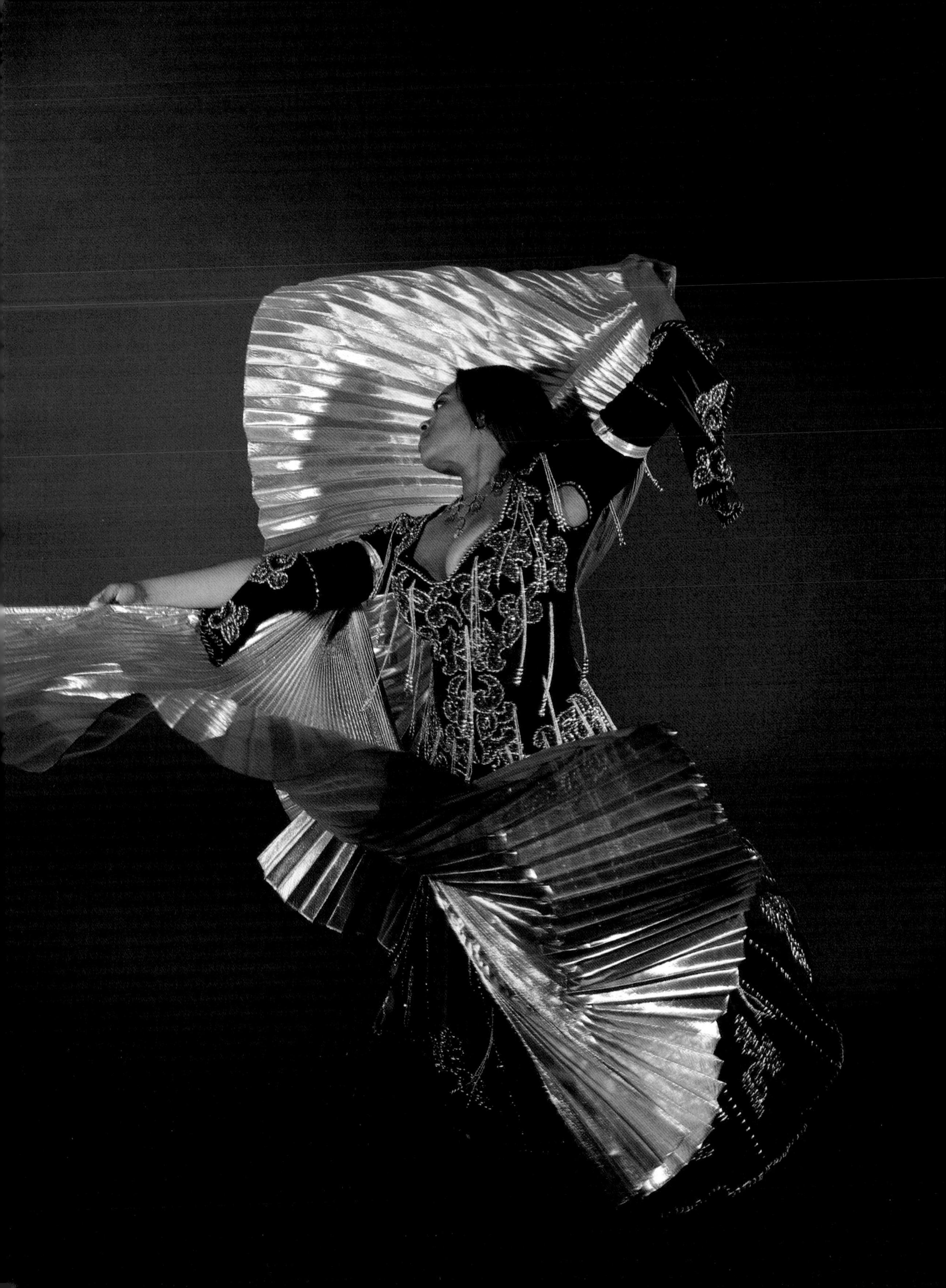

Introduction

"This above all; to thine own self be true."
WILLIAM SHAKESPEARE

By picking up this book you've confessed, at least to yourself, that at heart you are a romantic. I admitted the very same thing to myself years ago and like any romantic I am forever living in my imagination, in love with mystery, captivated by beauty, intoxicated with music, enraptured by emotion and obsessed with adventure. At the age of seven, I gazed upon the artefacts of King Tutankhamen's tomb on exhibit at the Smithsonian Museum. As I peered into the clear case that held the pharaoh's golden mask, I became hypnotized by its dazzling intricacy and subtle whispers of the past. From then on I was fascinated by ancient history – the grandeur of lost empires, the mysteries of the old world and the magic of the past.

I started belly dancing as a way to indulge my imagination while connecting with one of the lost eras that interested me most: the height of the Middle Eastern empire around the 1600s. That was a time in which tremendous strides were made in fields such as philosophy, medicine, art and poetry. Belly dancing seemed a delightful way to bring my interest in the ancient world into my very modern life. With its sensuous, feminine history, this art form was irresistible to me. I threw myself into its history and practice, and I hope, through this book, to share my enthusiasm with you.

The name belly dance is most likely derived from the French phrase *dance du ventre* or "dance of the stomach". Most modern dancers embrace this as an historical accuracy while others view it as a pejorative term created by tourists who made forays into the Middle East in the early 19th century. Belly dancing can also be referred to as "oriental dance", a title which covers both Middle Eastern and Near Eastern dance styles. Another name is *raks sharqui*, Arabic for "dance of the east". Although this term is primarily used to describe Egyptian cabaret style, it now has broader usage in America.

Dancing is a living, breathing element of human existence. Like all living things, it grows and changes with the world around it. Although it may not seem like it now, the roots of belly dancing are firmly entrenched in religious rituals focusing on goddess worship and/or fertility. Many ancient artefacts showing softly rounded women with large hips and breasts support anthropological theories promulgating the high status of women in archaic divinity structure because of their ability to give birth. The early pagan communities often worshipped a matriarchal deity and extolled the magic and fascination of the ability of women to create life. There is considerable historical evidence linking the ritualistic fertility dances of these cultures, which were symbolic re-creations of giving birth, to modern belly dancing. The sharp hip movements, deliberate muscular contractions and spasms, as well as sinewy undulations, demonstrate strong connections to the body's responses during labour and delivery.

But how did these rituals metamorphose into a form of mainstream public entertainment? The facts on this are limited and sketchy, but many people agree it was gypsy tribes who first drew dancing out into the street and developed it into theatre. The gypsies originally hailed from India and spoke in a Hindi-based language called Romany. Some time around the 5th century AD as a result of local oppression, need for work and sometimes banishment, the Romany gypsies began to migrate to other parts of the known world. Scholars suggest that many first travelled west into Afghanistan and Persia. From there, some migrated north to Turkey and on to Europe while others went south, following the coastline until they reached Egypt and other parts of North Africa. One of the ways that gypsies supported themselves during their nomadic journeys was by providing entertainment for the people of the communities in which they stopped.

The Romany left a cultural influence on many areas where they settled and the spell of their dance style remains strong in Central Asia, where Islamic communities have thrived for centuries. It is especially concentrated in Turkey and Egypt. The sophisticated religious belief structure of Islam had tremendous influence on all forms of entertainment and celebratory practice, dancing included. As a result of cultural segregation between the sexes, Muslim women were permitted only to be entertained by and celebrate with other women in closed quarters.

Belly dancing developed in different ways in each country the gypsies migrated through. In Turkey, after Fatih Sultan Mehmet II conquered Constantinople in 1453, the gypsies settled in the newly titled city of Istanbul. When entertainment was requested for the women, they were amused by female-only dancers and musicians called *chengis*. There are two theories for the origin of this name – the harp-like instrument called the *chang* or the Turkish word for gypsy, *chingene*. Working in organized groups, comprising the business leader, dancers and musicians, referred to as a *kol*, the *chengis* danced at bath houses, harems and other communal locations for women. They built an artistic style that is the root of many of the movements in belly dancing today. The complex hip work, shimmies and varied facial expressions, as well as veil dancing and finger cymbal playing, can be linked back to the gypsy *chengis,* who remained highly regarded and extremely popular until the end of the 19th century.

The strength of the dance form gradually failed when the power of the Ottoman Empire began to wane. Considerable economic collapse, social

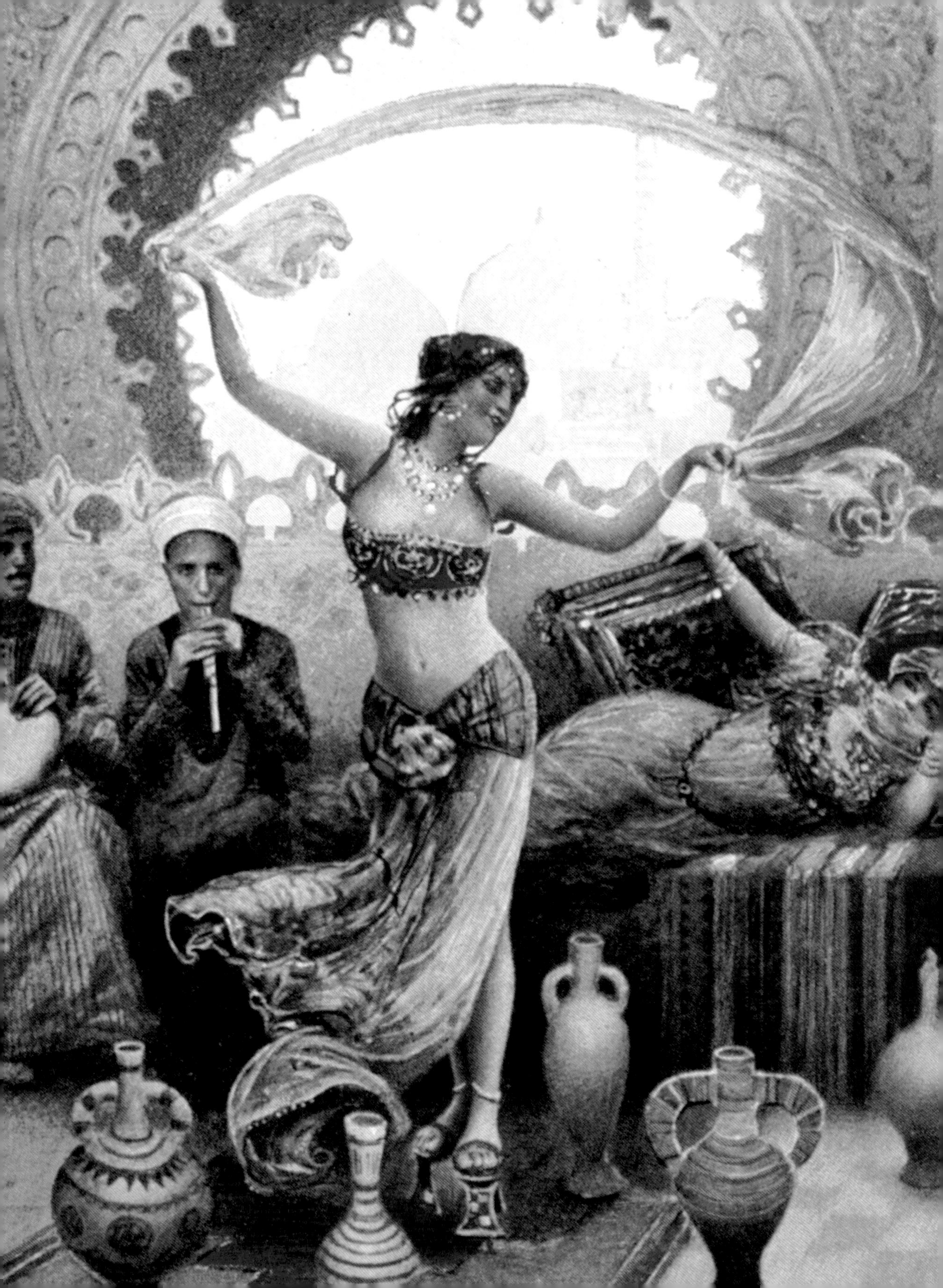

upheavals and modernizations ate away at the foundation of the *chengis* dancing troupes until what remained was a shadow of its former brilliance. In Turkey today, *chengis* dancing has become belly dancing and is primarily a tourist attraction, rather than secular entertainment.

As the gypsies continued their migration south into Egypt, the dancers were liberated for a time regarding their audiences. Performances were no longer exclusive to women. Gypsies also danced for the public at celebrations, wedding processions and in front of coffee houses and market places where the flow of people and money was greatest. Referred to as the *ghawazee*, their repertoire was a mix of music and dancing, including their own unique torso movements, native dances and improvised performances with veils, sticks, swords and candles. Some theorize that it was this public practice of dancing that generated the idea of adding coins to the performers' costume. As the gypsies danced, people who stopped to observe them would toss coins to their feet as tips. Without safe places to store their earnings, dancers sewed the money onto their clothes for safekeeping or used the coins to purchase jewellery which could always be worn.

Generally, public dancing was tolerated by the authorities because they earned a substantial revenue by taxing performers' profits. However, religious complaints and opinion finally outweighed the financial benefits, and public *ghawazee* dancing was outlawed in the city of Cairo in 1834.

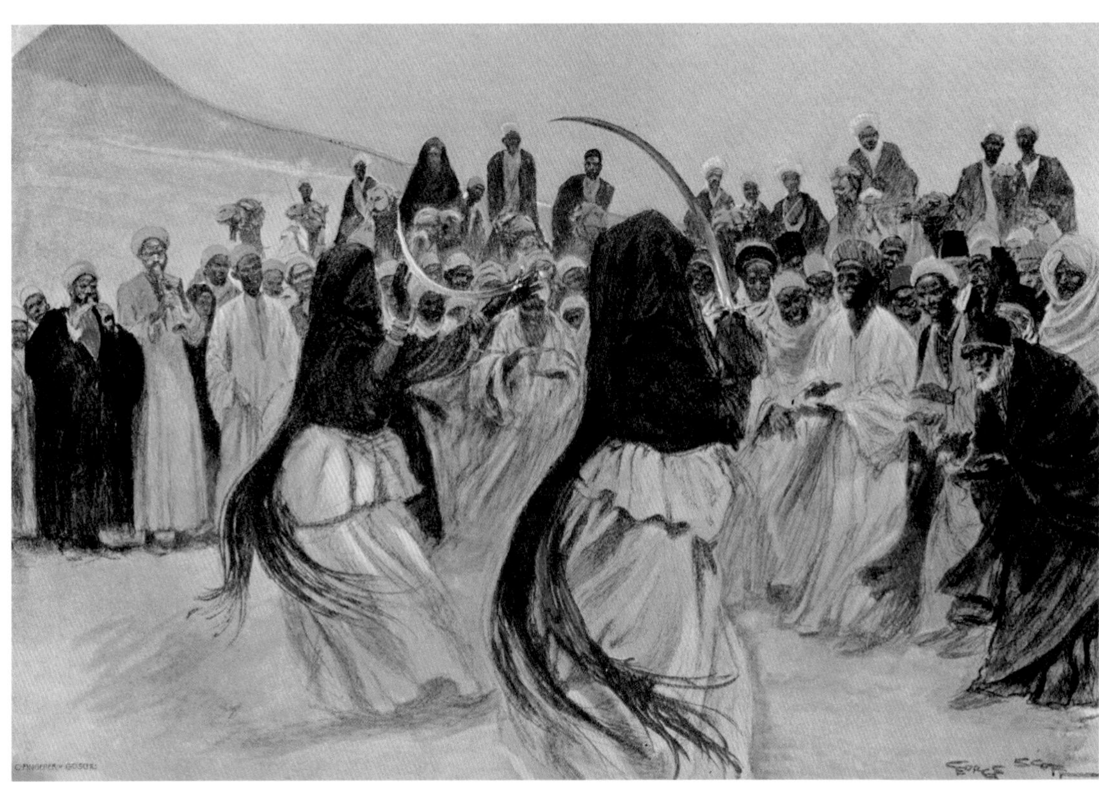

Punishments for breaking the edict were severe, including physical abuse for a first offence and years of hard labour for repeated offences, generally ending in banishment. At some point between 1849 and 1856, however, the ban was lifted and dancing was allowed to return to Cairo, although the sanction against dancing in public remained. The dance moved inside to a music-hall type environment and Egyptian cabaret-style dancing was born. At the turn of the century, it was given the name of belly dancing.

Belly dancing's expansion into Europe and America came from the ever-increasing flow of tourists into the Middle East. Dance troupes were contracted by foreigners and taken to exhibition forums in London, Paris and Chicago to perform their unique music and dancing. Their art was praised for its unique excitement – and condemned as lewd and scandalous because of its dramatic physical demonstrations. Belly dancing's popularity, even under this intense public scrutiny, remained undeniable and grew tenfold at the 1893 Chicago World's Fair with the publicity surrounding a belly dancer named Little Egypt. Reputedly of Syrian descent, Little Egypt sparked a wave of controversy. Her pelvic- and torso-focused dancing was imitated by so many to such an exaggerated extent that she began to protest against the impostors for distorting her performance into sheer vulgarity. This is one of the earliest examples of belly dancing being twisted into overt public sexuality from its more subtle origins.

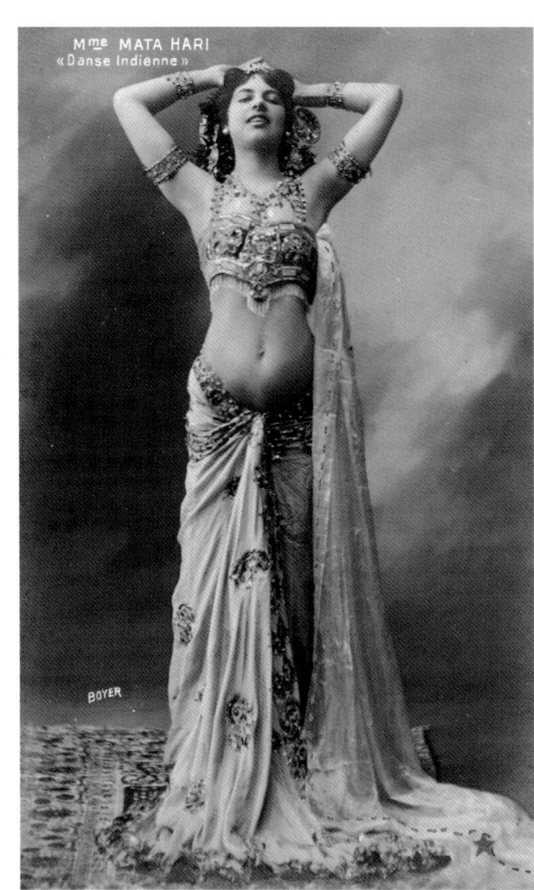

The fantasized and often distorted version of belly dancing grew at a rapid pace, becoming a popular subject in books, art and Hollywood movies. Its image dominated by the burlesque temptress style fed to us by a sex-hungry entertainment industry, belly dancing was not something that appealed to most of the female population. But in recent years more and more women have discovered the true elements of this incredibly feminine and self-affirming art form. By combining the best of the ancient and the modern, contemporary belly dancers have been able to rejuvenate the dance from the taints of yesterday to the visual delight of today, appealing to people of all ages and backgrounds.

It is with dedicated love for and appreciation of belly dancing that I write this book. I hope that it brings you on a journey through history as well as acting as an inspiring passage to your inner spirit – and a way to express it to yourself and the world.

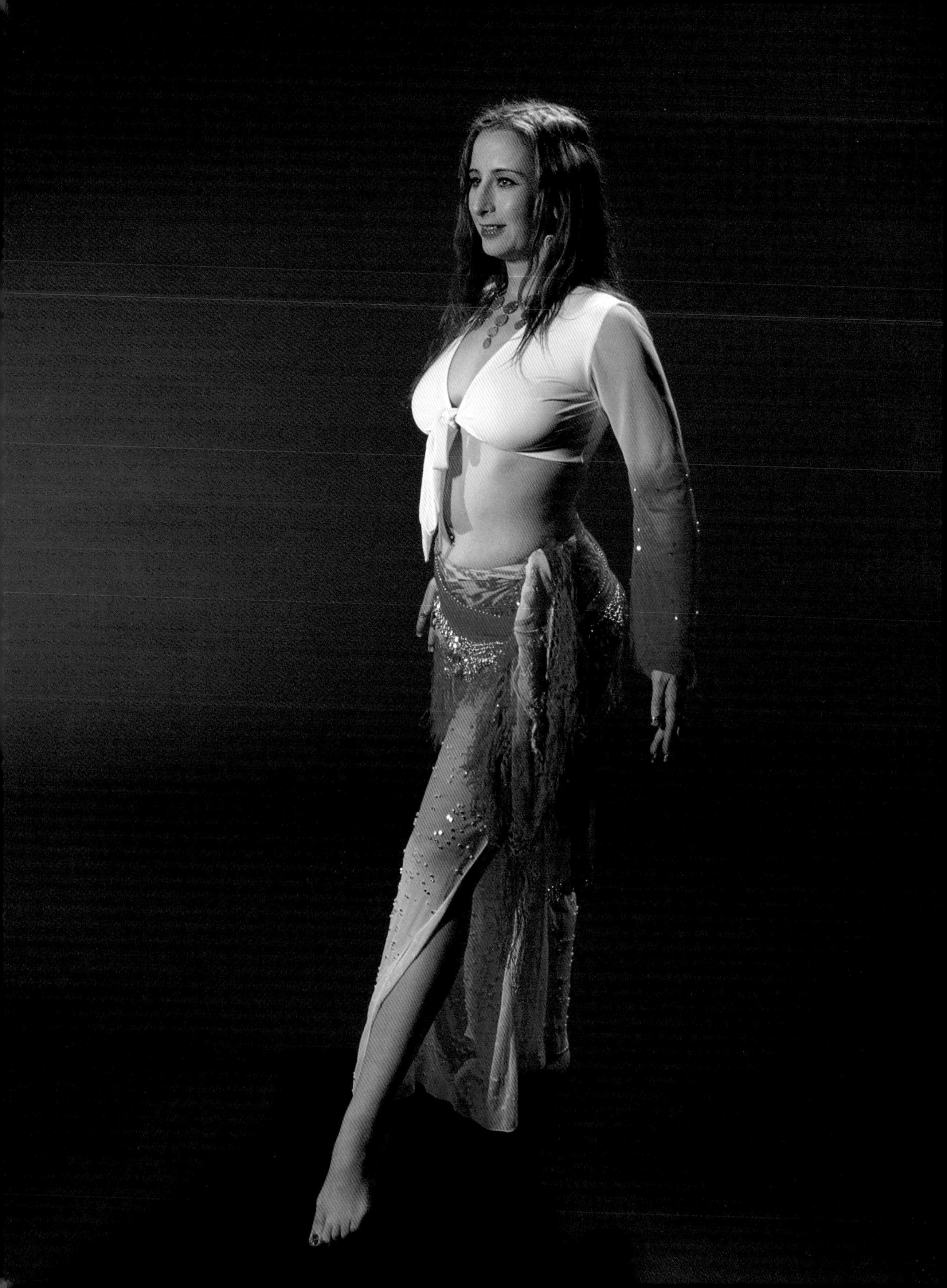

1 Getting started

Learning to belly dance has almost unlimited benefits and you will feel improvements in both your physical and mental wellbeing soon after you start. On a spiritual level, belly dancing promotes a positive body image. Today's fashion is for an almost emaciated thinness which borders on the unhealthy and can have negative physiological effects. Low body weight can affect mood, increase stress on the heart, disrupt the sleep cycle and deregulate normal gland functioning. It may also be linked to erratic menstrual cycles. Just think – a woman's desire to be supermodel-thin might damage one of the quintessential aspects of being female! Few women are born with the build and metabolism to achieve the current popular body image, leaving a very hard and disappointing road for others, who strive to measure up but cannot because of their natural shape.

Belly dancing is a wonderful way to counteract these negative body images and celebrate the more natural, curvaceous feminine form in all its shapes and sizes. In the ancient world, when belly dancing came into being, thinness was a sign of poverty, sickness and starvation. For a woman of those times, having a soft layer surrounding her bones showed that she was well fed and healthy, possessed financial means and was endowed with security and happiness. Remember that when you look at your body in the mirror!

Most people are more open to learning when they feel relaxed and comfortable and this is certainly true for belly dancing. One of the best things about belly dancing is that you can really let yourself go, physically and mentally. The easiest way to facilitate this release is to take a few moments to create a good space where you can dance.

CREATING A POSITIVE DANCE ENVIRONMENT

If you are at home, find somewhere that allows about 2m (6ft) of space all round your central point. The measurements don't have to be exact, but you need enough room to move with as little restriction as possible. You should also have a large mirror in front of you in which you can see yourself from about 60cm (2ft) above your head down to your toes.

Privacy is important, particularly when you first start. Dancing in the daylight which streams through your windows during the day is a delight, but this does expose you to the curious eyes of passers-by. However, if you drape lengths of sheer fabric in a variety of colours over your window you will have the benefits of natural light, tinted into different hues, while protecting your dance retreat from the gaze of others. You can buy extremely inexpensive polyester chiffon in any colour which takes your fancy from your local fabric shop.

This simple technique can be used in the evening as well. When dancing after sunset, low, soft lighting is preferable to the hard glare of fluorescents. If you do not have a dimmer switch, cover your lights with lengths of dark-hued sheer fabrics.

Day or night, scented candles are a delightful addition to your setting. Use a variety of candles on candlesticks and in bowls and glasses to add a soothing and mysterious atmosphere to your dance space. Some dancers prefer to use the heady scent of burned patchouli or sandalwood incense to create a spiritual dance space. Incense sticks or cones are perfect. Just make sure you have the right burner so you avoid burns or fire. Others like to anoint their pulse points with earthy musky oils so that when they start to move, their body heat causes the fragrance to be released.

The aim when creating positive space at home is to build a spiritually warm atmosphere, which brings you emotional contentment and security. However, if you prefer to practice in a professional studio, look for one that has windows with full shade coverage and a floor made of varnished hard wood which is smooth to the touch. The surroundings should be clean and without obstacles.

WHAT TO WEAR

Next, think about proper dress for dancing. There is a wonderful variety of clothing for belly dancing beyond the costumes you see on professionals wearing. Whatever you wear to dance in, try to find something that matches the following requirements.

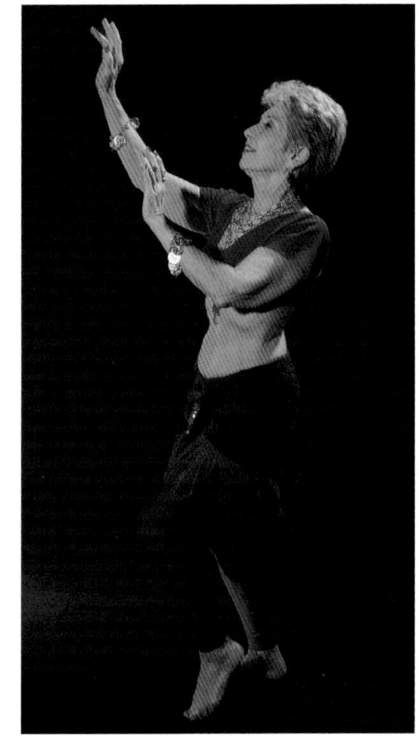

• Choose something that does not restrict your movement in any way. Freedom of body expression is essential to good belly dancing. Beginners often feel most comfortable in a sports bra top. These special tops are made for exercises that are more demanding than beginning belly dance and are ideal for supporting your breasts, while allowing freedom for your arms and shoulders and leaving your midriff visible. Other options are shelf bra tank tops or cotton yoga shirts folded up above your midriff.

• Be brave and allow for a top that fully exposes your midsection. No matter how big or small, you don't have to be shy – allow your belly and hips to show. No holding back now! For your legs, a pair of lightweight running or yoga tights rolled over at the waist down to your hip bones is a great inexpensive choice.

- Find something light and feminine such as a gypsy-style shawl or silk scarves to drape round your hips.

Once you get into belly dancing you might like to invest in practice clothing to make you look the part. There are plenty of wonderful belly dance clothes to choose from which will make you feel like you just stepped out of an Oriental painting. Try costume-type bra tops, vest tops, cholis and tie-arounds for your upper body. Underneath, flowing harem pants and billowy gypsy skirts give unlimited range of movement and feeling.

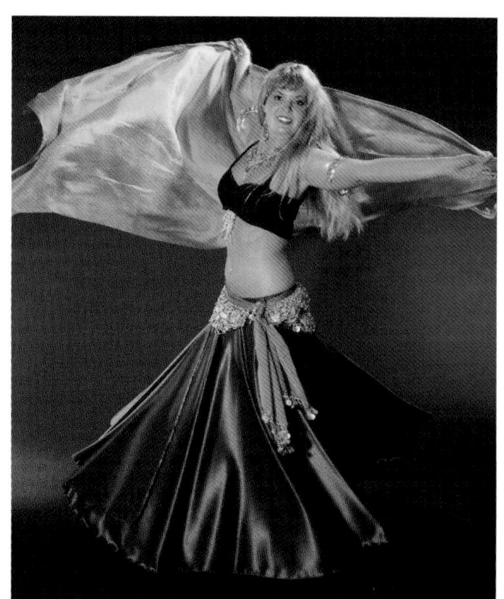

Coin belts come in every colour and design you can think of and are worth every penny for the fun they add to your dancing. When purchasing, give the coin belt a good shake to see how loud the coins ring. The louder, the better! This exciting jingling adds incredible spirit and authenticity to the dance and can spark your imagination like nothing else.

RELAX YOUR MIND AND BODY

To bring yourself into the right frame of mind and lift your spirits, start with some breathing exercises to relax your mind and body and release tension.

- Stand or sit comfortably and close your eyes.
- Relax your abdominal muscles and inhale deeply for five heartbeats. Let your stomach extend fully so you draw in as much air as possible.
- When five beats are up, hold the air in your lungs for two beats and then release your breath completely for another six beats. You should feel your shoulders and neck muscles relaxing.
- Repeat this exercise at least four times. If you are feeling particularly tense, repeat the breathing technique until you feel calm and peaceful.

Imagination is a powerful tool that will also help you get into the right frame of mind. There is inspiration everywhere and it is always helpful to conjure up a romantic image that helps drain away daily stress. While you are practising your breathing, let your imagination take you somewhere magical. My favourite phrase in belly dancing is "anything is possible".

Maybe your mind will take you to a simple flower garden with cool grass under your feet, or to a white sandy beach with the ocean lapping the shore. My personal favourite is to imagine myself in a desert oasis in the early evening, with a cool and gentle breeze flowing over me. Wherever you wish to go at that moment is fine.

SELECTING MUSIC

The music of the Middle East has incredible soul and touches upon all aspects of human emotion. Whatever you are feeling, from joy and sadness to ecstasy and surprise, you can find music to match your mood. The most common instruments in Middle Eastern music are the *oud*, the *nay*, the *kunoon* and the *dumbek*. To the dancer, however, the most important of these instruments is the *dumbek*, or drum. It establishes the tempo of the music and by following the rhythm of the drum, you can establish the proper pace for dancing.

The single best tool a dancer has to keep her dancing in time with her music is what she learned in primary school – counting from one to eight! As you practice the techniques in this book, count out loud to the beats in the music. When your timing skills improve, you can start counting in your head instead of out loud. This is a simple technique, but unfortunately, many dancers, once they feel they have mastered counting, give up on it. This nearly always leads to sloppy technique. The strongest dancers keep counting no matter what level of expertise they reach.

In the early stages of dancing, the easiest way to find the beat is by marching to it. Simply step from left to right, tapping each foot when you hear the sound of the *dumbek* drum. There are some inspiring popular rhythms in traditional music which are helpful for a beginning belly dancer to get to know.

The traditional eight-count beat is the simplest and is basically eight uniform beats sounded one after another:
(one two three four five six seven eight)
Doom doom doom doom doom doom doom doom
● ● ● ● ● ● ● ●

Another popular rhythm is the *chiftitelli*. It is so closely associated with the Middle East that even people who aren't interested in Arabic music will recognize it:
(one twothree fourfive six seven eight)
Doom doomdoom doomdoom dom dom dom
● ●● ●● ● ● ●

The *moqsoom*, mostly used for creative hip work, is very simple:
(onetwo pause three pause onetwo pause three)
Domdom dom domdom dom
●● ● ●● ●

A very advanced rhythm that has its origins in Turkey and Greece is the complex nine/eight rhythm. The nine/eight is an amazing musical annotation that is very rapid and energetic:
(one two three four five six SEVEN eight nine)
Doom doom doom doom doom doom DOOMdom doom

SUGGESTED ALBUMS FOR BELLY DANCING

When you first start belly dancing, the music and artists will be unfamiliar to you. Beginners risk spending lots of money on music only to find that its unsuitable for dancing. To avoid this, I've chosen some musicians and albums with excellent music for the beginner.

TURKISH: OMAR FARUK TEKBILEK
Gypsy Fire
Crescent Moon
Dance into Eternity
Firedance

ETHNIC COMPILATIONS: GEORGE ABDO
Best of Bellydance from Egypt, Lebanon, Arabia and Turkey

EGYPTIAN: HOSSAM RAMSEY
Source of Fire
Rhythms of the Nile
Secrets of the Eye

MODERN/POP BELLY DANCE MUSIC
Natasha Atlas: *Halim*
Alabina: *The Voice of Alabina*
Amr Diab: *The Best of Amr Diab*

NEW AGE BELLY DANCE MUSIC
Jehan Kamal: *Serpent Rising*
Azam Ali: *Portals of Grace*
Vas: *In the Garden of Souls*

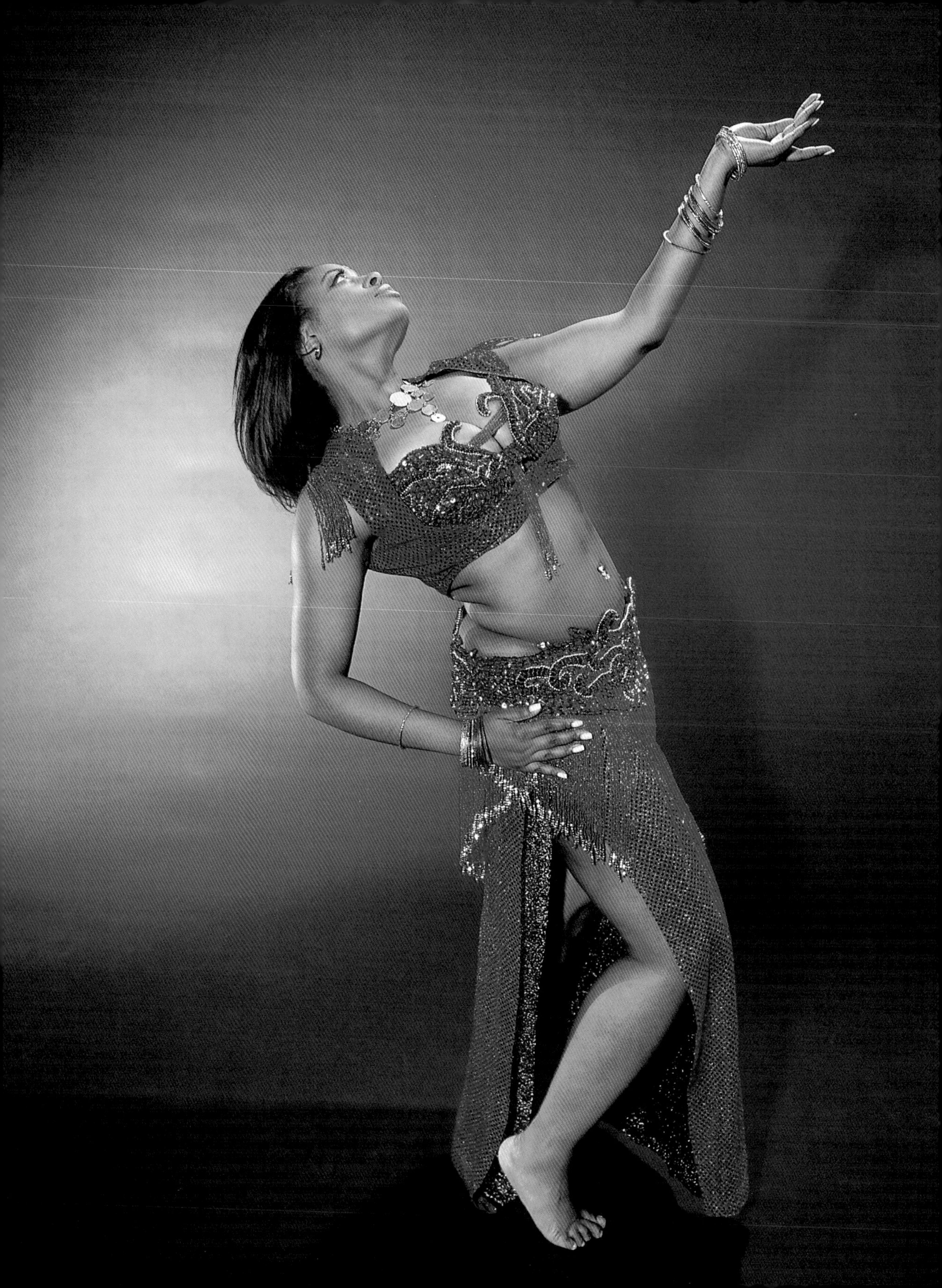

2 Preparation

With any form of instruction I believe that it is vital for a student to learn each element of the new skill correctly the first time it's taught. First impressions stick with you. When something is learned properly the first time, it's remembered that way for life. Each type of dance has its own foundation of techniques which beginners must understand and master before they can move on, and belly dancing is no exception. The four most important skills for the beginner to learn are primary dance counting, weight distribution, muscle isolation and correct body posture (p.20).

DANCE COUNTING

Every dancer must follow the technique of counting, especially in the beginning. Belly dance music has a wide range of complex rhythms, but the best one for learning is a simple eight-count beat – the drum or underlying rhythm repeats every eight beats. With that in mind, for the dance steps to operate in time with the music, a count of eight is used to monitor and manage every step at all times. Each step and each move are given a count or set of counts that will total eight beats.

WEIGHT DISTRIBUTION

Each step we take – walking, running, dancing or even skipping – is accompanied by shifts in body weight. When you are dancing, understanding your body weight and where it is held will bring an improvement in grace and balance. As we stand still, our weight is evenly distributed, with 50 percent on each side. If the right knee is bent, our weight naturally shifts to the left side to offset the lack of balance on the right. If the left leg is lifted up off the ground, then 100 percent of the weight is supported by the right leg.

To help understand this concept, place your right foot in front of your left and sway your upper body back and forth in a rocking motion. Feel how your body shifts the weight backward and forward to maintain balance. In the foundation position (p.20), note that when you lean back, 70 percent of your weight will be on your back leg while 30 percent is on your front leg.

MUSCLE ISOLATION

Isolation is the term dancers use to describe the act of intentionally moving only one part of the body at a time, while keeping the other parts still and relaxed. In other words, you isolate the muscles that you want to use and freeze those you're not using. Isolation helps develop your muscles properly during practice for stronger and more distinct movements.

PROPER POSTURE: THE FOUNDATION

Stand with your feet 30cm (12in) apart and parallel, knees unlocked. Straighten your spine until there is not even the slightest slouch in your upper body. Gently push your shoulders back and lift your chin to a comfortable level, about 1cm (½in) higher than normal. Flex your abdominal muscles until your stomach is slightly lifted and you feel tension in your lower abdomen. You body should appear calm but proud.

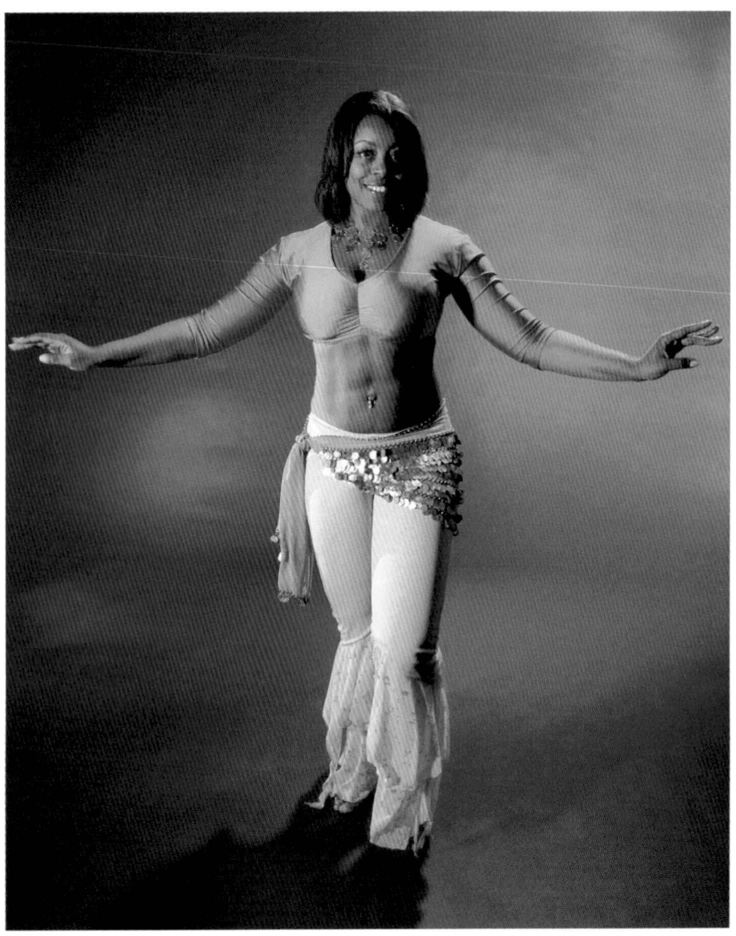

UPPER BODY

Having your arms in the proper position makes the difference between looking graceful and looking awkward. With your arms bent slightly at the elbow, raise them at your sides until your hands are about chest level. Bend your wrists, just slightly raising your hands.

LOWER BODY

Bend your knees just a little so that they are soft, then slide your left foot 15cm (6in) forward. Rise up onto the ball of your left foot, arching your heel sharply upward. Take a moment to note your weight distribution. At first, many people stand in this posture with 50 percent of their weight on each foot. In this position, 70 percent of the body weight should be on the back leg, and 30 percent on the front. If you are standing with a 50/50 distribution, lean back slightly and your weight will naturally shift onto the back leg. Don't lean all the way back – just enough to transfer more than half your weight to your back leg.

HAND POSITIONS

There are two basic hand positions – both are easy to achieve, yet look elegant. These positions help you learn how to hold your hands beautifully, without distracting from what the rest of your body is doing.

BASIC 1: THE BASIC HAND

Keeping your wrist arched, straighten your right hand until it is sharp and tense. Hold for a few moments, then slightly relax so there is a softness in the joints. Slightly raise your little finger and forefinger while dropping your middle finger and thumb.

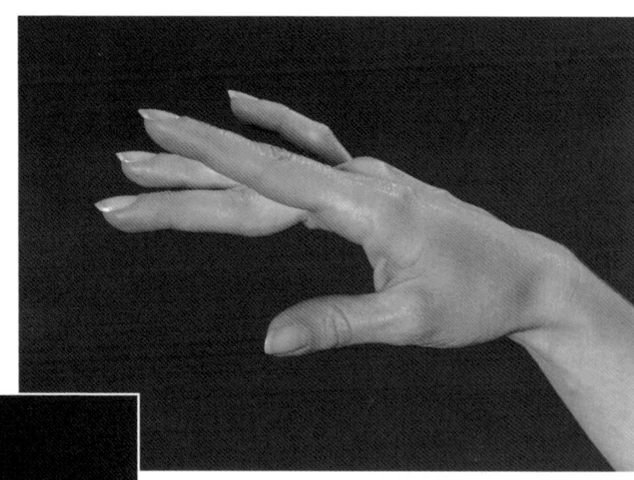

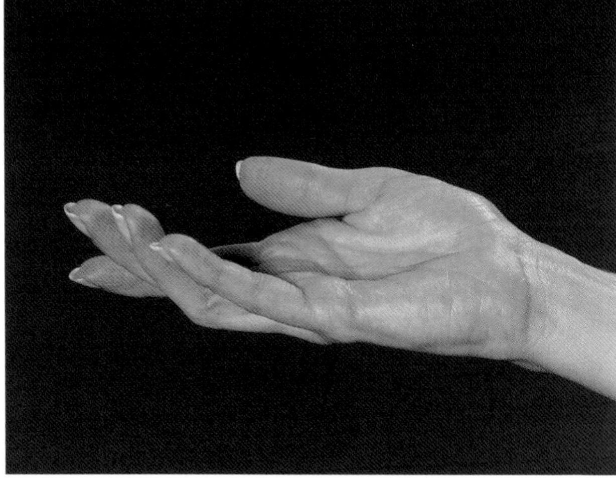

BASIC 2: THE OFFERING HAND

Hold out your hand with the palm and forearm facing upward. Starting with the little finger, allow your fingers to curl up very slightly while keeping your forefinger almost perfectly straight.

STRETCH AND WARM UP

Before any physical activity, it is important to stretch and warm up your body to prevent injury as well as soreness. It's also easier to achieve the natural movements of belly dancing after some gentle stretches. Practice these stretches daily and your flexibility – and your dancing – will improve.

NECK STRETCH

Begin by slowly rolling your head right round in a circle. Roll four times to the left and four to the right.

1 Keeping your left arm and shoulder relaxed, take your right hand and reach it over your crown. Rest your fingertips over your left ear and breathe in. When you breathe out, gently pull your head down and to the right. Make sure you don't lift your left shoulder. Take two breaths, feeling your neck muscles uncoil, and release.

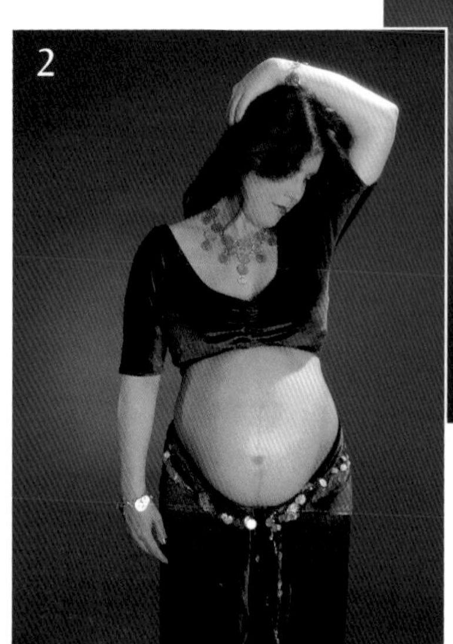

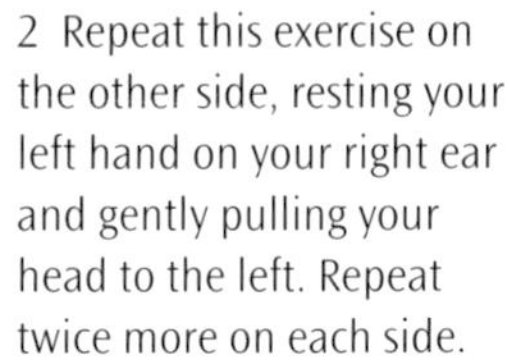

2 Repeat this exercise on the other side, resting your left hand on your right ear and gently pulling your head to the left. Repeat twice more on each side.

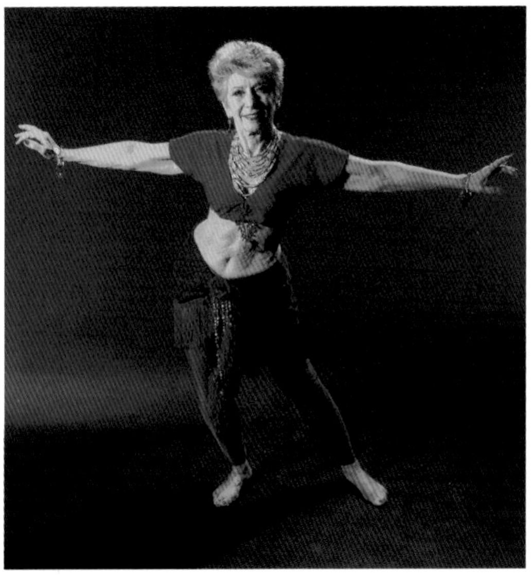

HIP-RELEASING STRETCH

Stand with your feet shoulder-width apart and raise your arms out to your sides. Keeping your feet flat on the ground, bend your knees and gently push your hips as far as you can to the right. Try almost to sit without falling over, as though you're balancing the littlest part of your cheek on a stool while still supporting yourself with your legs! Hold this position for ten seconds and breathe. You will feel your hip joints starting to pull and release.

Return to the center and stretch to your left side, again holding for ten seconds.

Repeat twice more. Speed up by shifting all the way out to the left and right in one fluid movement, gently bouncing once or twice on each side.

BACK-RELEASING STRETCH

The hip and torso movements in belly dancing use the muscles that encircle your pelvis and run down your lower back. Stretching these muscles before you practice will help you develop flexibility and strength, and improve the quality of your dancing.

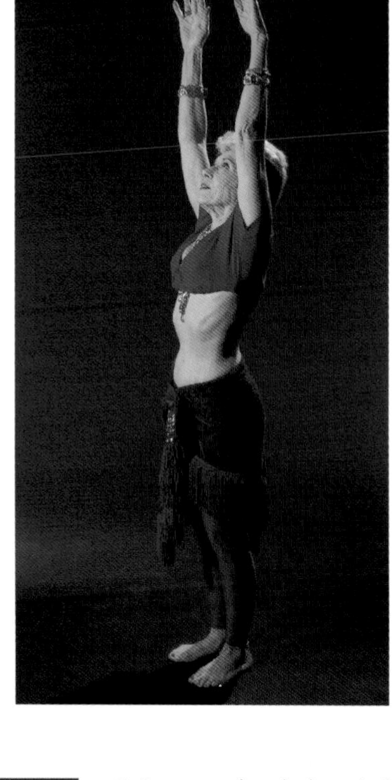

1 Stand with your feet parallel and raise both arms straight up above your head. Keep your shoulders pressed down.

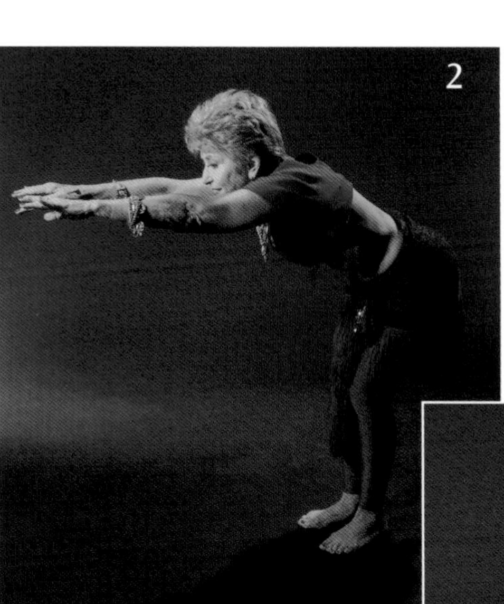

2 Slowly bend forward with a flat back (don't curl down), hinging at the waist and gently bending your knees until your torso is parallel with the floor.

3 Drop your hands down in front of you and touch the floor. If you cannot touch the floor, gently bend your knees and simply reach as far as is comfortable for you. Take a deep breath and relax. When you are supported by your hands, flex and release your knees a few times on each side in a walking motion.

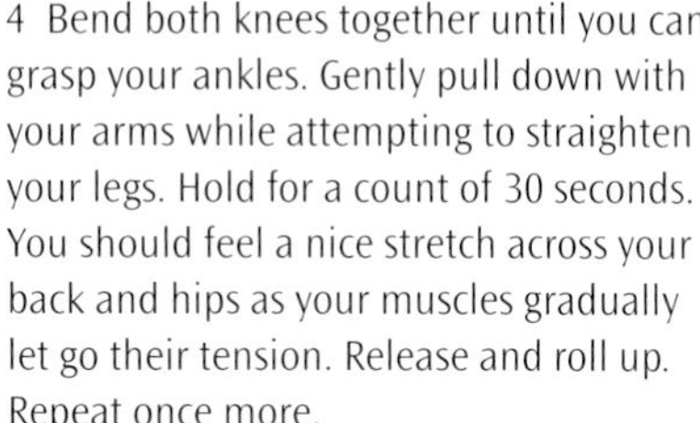

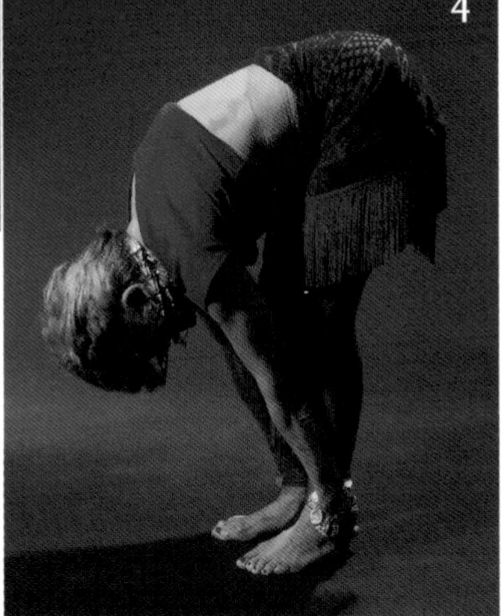

4 Bend both knees together until you can grasp your ankles. Gently pull down with your arms while attempting to straighten your legs. Hold for a count of 30 seconds. You should feel a nice stretch across your back and hips as your muscles gradually let go their tension. Release and roll up. Repeat once more.

HAMSTRING STRETCH

This stretch will help to loosen tight hamstrings and calf muscles. Don't force your muscles. If you cannot reach your ankles, just gently stretch as far as you can. You know your body best, and it's the only one you have, so be careful with it!

1 Take a wide step to your left so that your feet are about 1.2m (4ft) apart. Stretch out your arms, reaching from your shoulders as though you're trying to touch the walls. Feel your shoulder blades begin to release. Slowly bend forward with a flat back (don't curl down), hinging at the waist while gently bending your knees until your torso is horizontal with the floor.

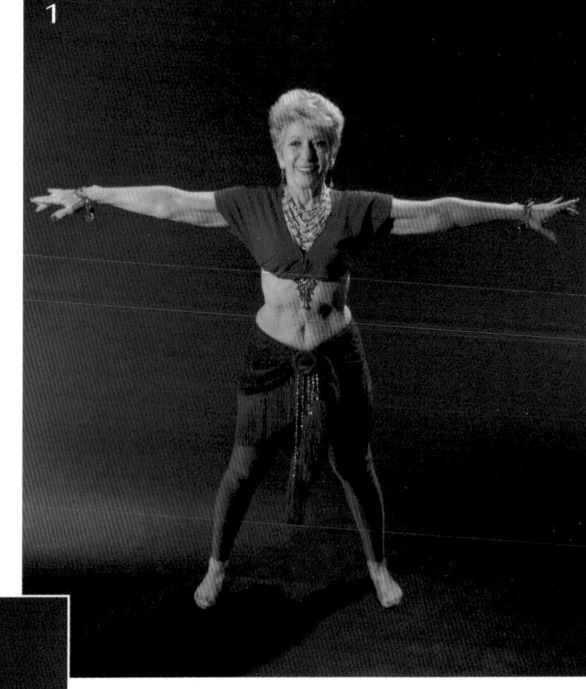

1

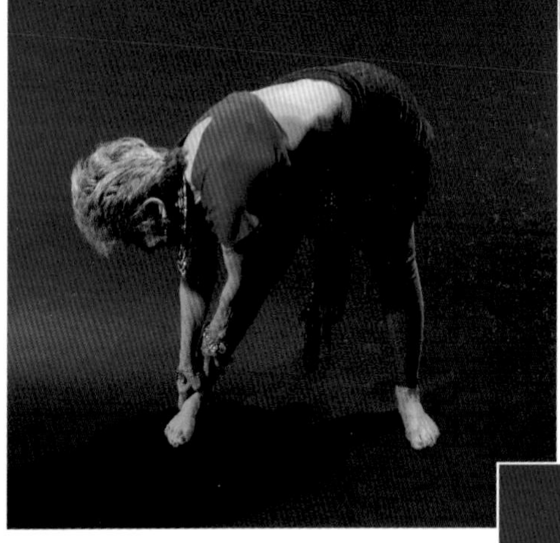

2

2 Rotate your body to the right and reach down with both hands to grasp your right ankle. Take a deep breath in. As you breathe out, pull gently on your ankle, bringing your lower body down for 20 seconds and allowing your calf and hamstring muscles to release. Rise up and repeat the stretch on the other side.

3 When you've stretched both sides, return to the center. Drop directly down, reaching as far as you can toward both your ankles. Grasp them firmly. Breathe in and as you breathe out, gently pull on your ankles and allow your hip muscles to release. Repeat all the stretches.

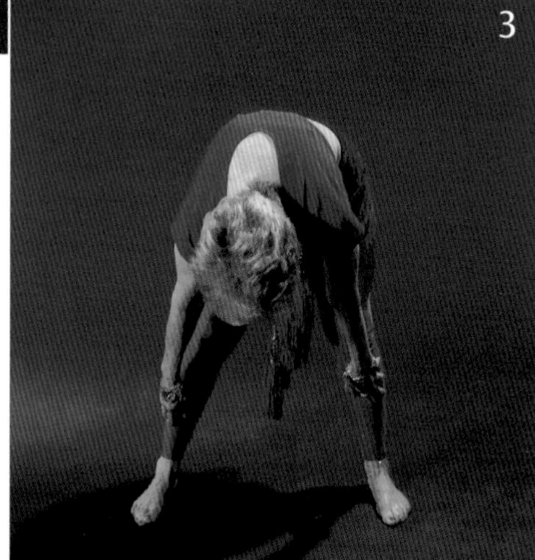

3

WRIST-RELEASING STRETCH

Graceful hands are important in belly dancing, so keep your wrists supple with this stretch.

1 With palms together, hold your hands at chest level.

2 Press your palms together and lower your arms until your hands are at abdomen level. Make sure you keep your lower palms touching. Hold for a count of five. Repeat twice.

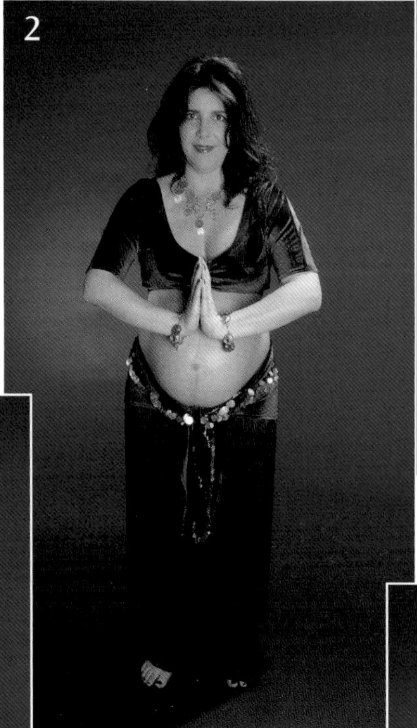

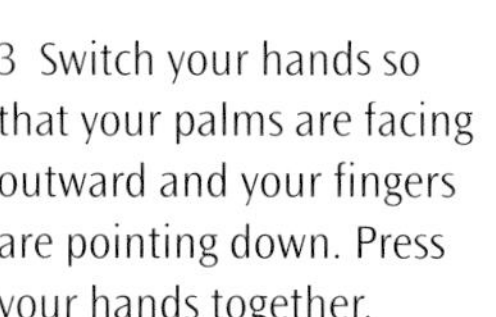

3 Switch your hands so that your palms are facing outward and your fingers are pointing down. Press your hands together.

4 Gently drop your elbows down to lift your wrists slightly until you feel a stretch in your forearms. Hold for a count of five. Repeat twice.

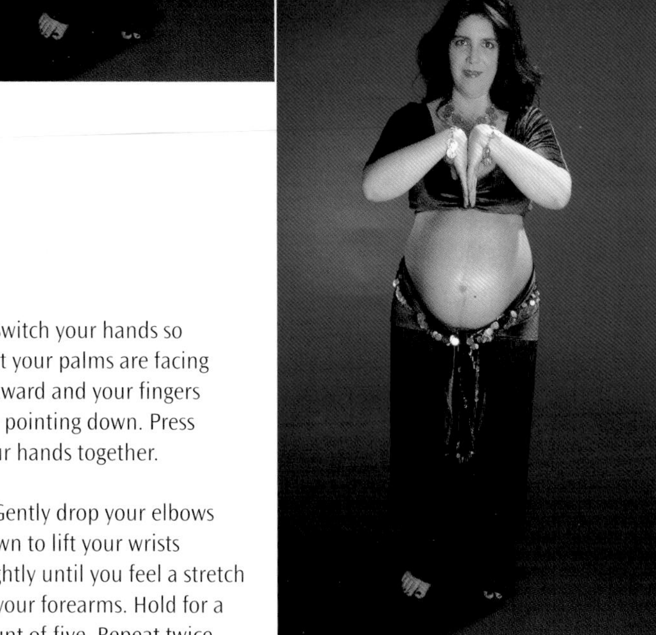

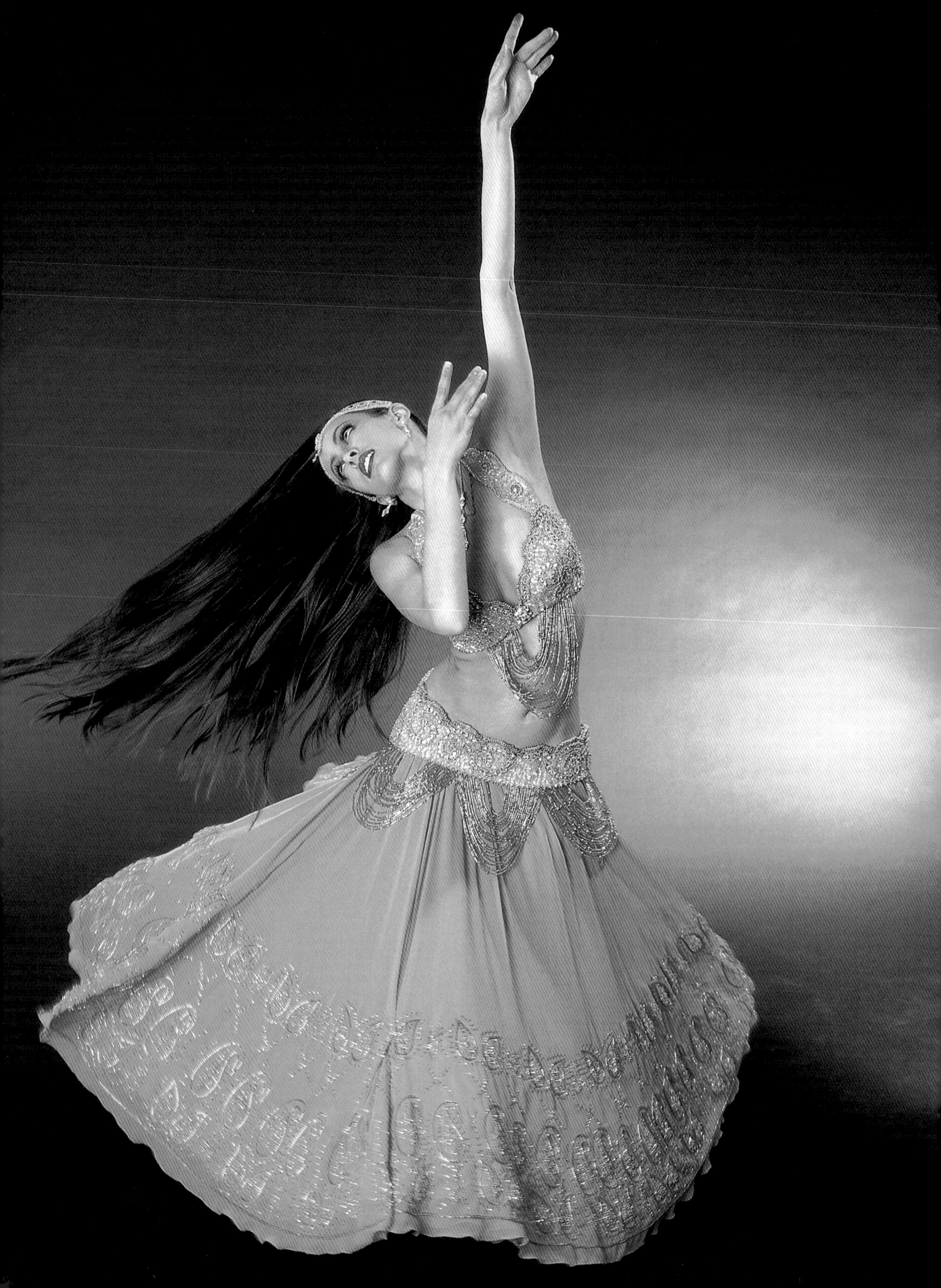

3 Basic elements

When you were a child you had to learn to walk before you could run. Before walking, you had to learn to stand, and before standing came crawling. The truth is, belly dancing is no different! Dedicating time and patience to the measured and steady progression of your abilities is the best way to learn the basic movements on the following pages. These steps make up the primary vocabulary of beginner belly dance and it is vital to master them before leaping into more complex motions.

When finding your way through the instructions, try not to skim over movements that come easily to you. Rather, practice them and focus on understanding why your body responds so well to those particular physical patterns. This knowledge will help if you reach a stumbling block with another movement. Should this happen, don't get frustrated – be patient and allow yourself time to think through the step, grasping each component, then putting the movement together.

As you grow more comfortable with the steps, I urge you to experiment and improvise. Try alternating between fast and slow as you practice, noting how the contrast changes the steps. Vary the level of energy you put into the movements, performing some with sharp, muscular jerks and others with soft and gentle fluidity. You'll be amazed at the difference these easy changes will make in all your basic (and later more complex) practice movements.

Turning and spinning (pp.65–69) are especially delightful to experiment with, but a bit more tricky. Have you ever seen a professional dancer turn and turn and never appear to get dizzy? That is because of the technique called "spotting". To spot, look straight ahead and focus on a single point in front of you. Turn round as far as you can without removing your eyes from that point. When you can't turn any further, quickly spin your head round with the turn to look over the other shoulder. Locate the original point you focused on until your body catches up. Repeat this five times quickly. Now spin five times without spotting. Feel the difference? No matter how fast/slow or sharp/smooth your movements, spotting will spare you many swimming heads and stumbles.

Simple as these steps may seem, when put together in artful combinations, they can be used to build stunning dances and routines. While adding more and more steps to your dance vocabulary, really allow yourself to play around by "layering" them. That means taking the separate techniques and layering one on top of the other to develop a string of movements that add up to a dance. Layering is truly where the fun begins – by applying it, your skills will develop from the simplicity of a planned series of steps to joyfully intricate, spontaneous dancing.

HIP DROPS

This is the ideal step for learning how to move and isolate your hips and a very important movement in belly dancing.

1 First double check that your body is in a strong foundation position with proper weight distribution (p.20).

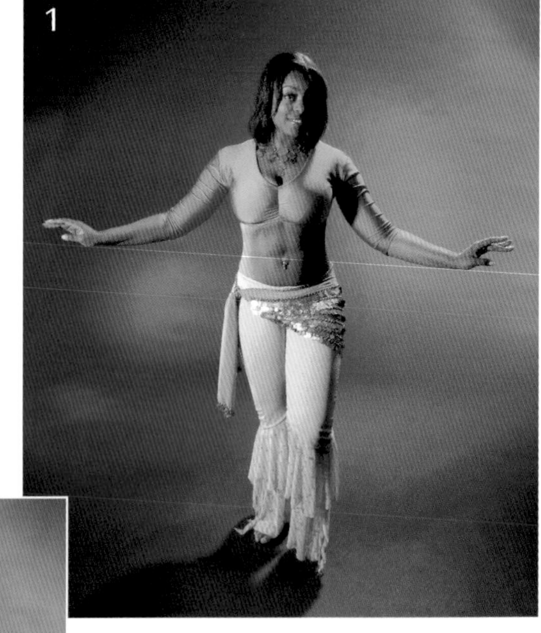
1

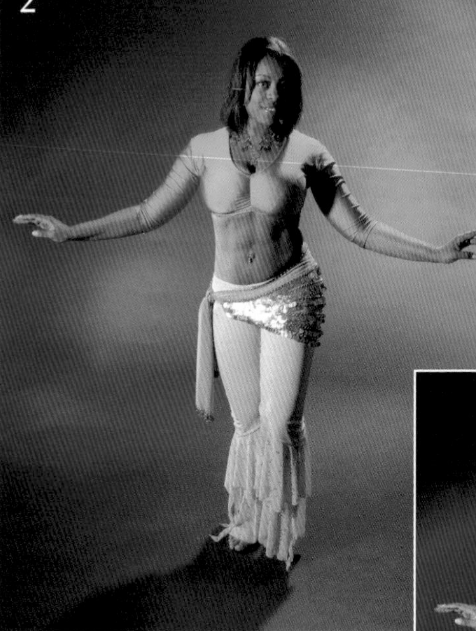
2

2 Lift your left hip slowly by contracting the muscles that run down the left side of your abdomen. As you lift your hip, don't lift the rest of you! Keep your head in an even position by allowing your left knee to bend a little and your right to straighten slightly, while pulling your hip up.

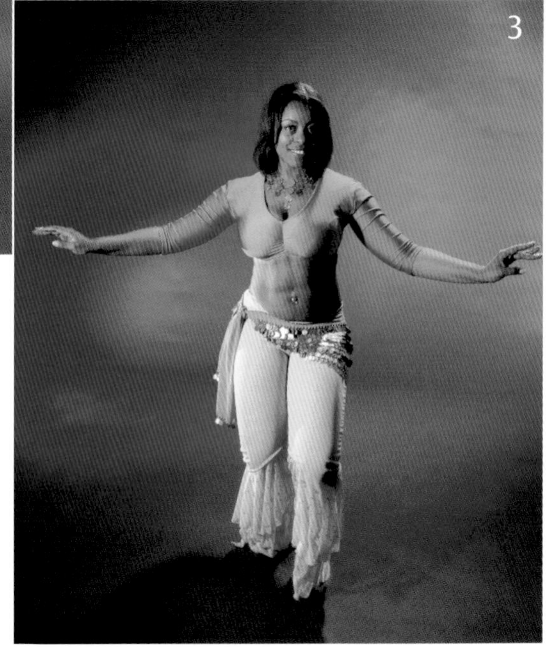
3

3 When your hip is as high as it can go, hold it there for two counts, then drop it sharply by releasing the contraction and actively using your leg and pelvic strength to force the hip down lower than its original position in foundation. Hold it there for another two counts, accentuating the down motion. Raise the hip slowly, again counting one, two in your head, and sharply drop it while counting three, four. Repeat on your right side.

HIP LIFTS

This a simple variation of the hip drop. During the hip drop, the down/dropping motion is accentuated. In a lift, it is the opposite – the upward motion is accentuated.

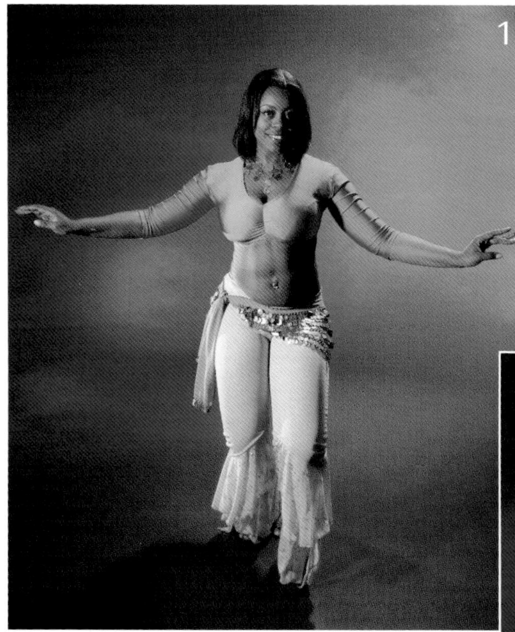

1 Starting in foundation position (p.20) and using the same count speed as the hip drop, sharply lift your hip with a jerk.

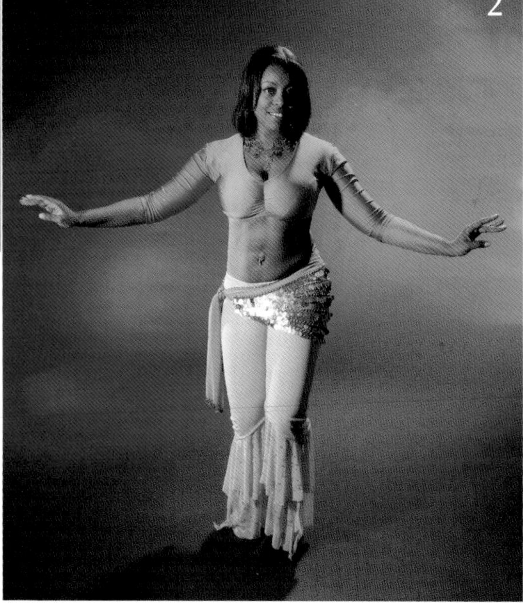

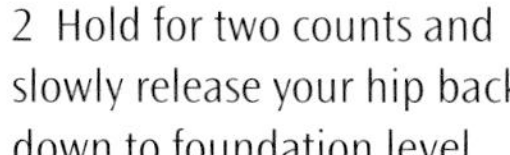

2 Hold for two counts and slowly release your hip back down to foundation level.

PRACTICE

Perform ten hip lifts on the right and ten on the left. Speed up so that it only takes one count to lift your hip and one count to drop it for another ten lifts.

PRACTICING THE HIP LIFT AND HIP DROP TOGETHER

Using two counts, practice 20 hip drops on the left and 20 on the right. Then repeat, but using only one count per hip drop. Switch to high and low hip drops for 20 on each side. Finally, transition into hip lifts by completing a hip drop, holding it for one beat, then moving quickly into a hip lift. Remember, for hip lifts and drops to look as they should, always accentuate the drop or lift with a brisk, sharp movement and keep the opposing release soft.

HIP SNAPS AND HIP THRUSTS

These moves may look simple, but to master them you must be able to control your hip muscles while relaxing your knees, to allow your hips more range.

LEFT AND RIGHT HIP SNAP

1 As you stand in foundation (p.20), bend your supporting leg 7.5cm (3in) more than usual. Increasing the bend on the supporting leg gives your hips more room to move. In one fast movement, bend your right leg down, straighten your left leg slightly and sharply snap your left hip out to the left.

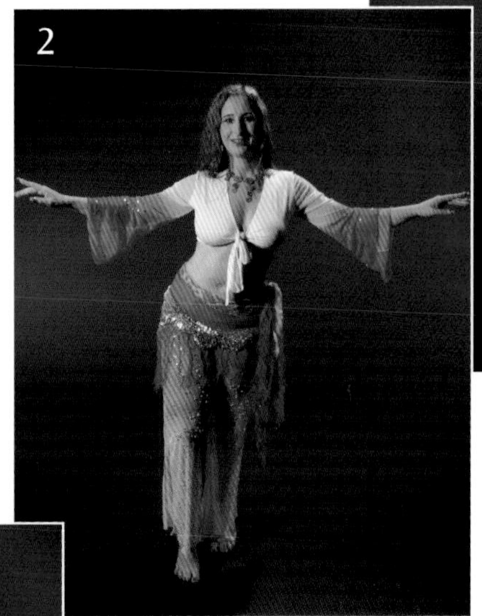

2 Then quickly bend your left leg down, straighten your right and sharply snap your right hip out to the right. Alternate left and right in short sharp movements until you've done ten snaps on each side. Each snap should equal one count.

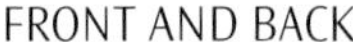

FRONT AND BACK

3 Now, just as fast as with the left and right snap, softly bend your knees and snap your pelvis a little to the front by tightening your abdomen muscles sharply. A small fast snap is enough – any more can look vulgar.

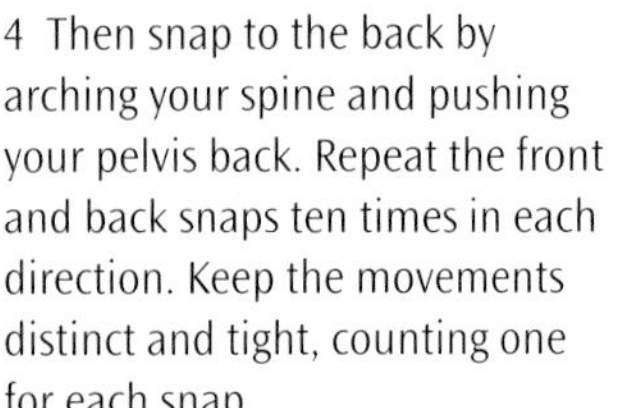

4 Then snap to the back by arching your spine and pushing your pelvis back. Repeat the front and back snaps ten times in each direction. Keep the movements distinct and tight, counting one for each snap.

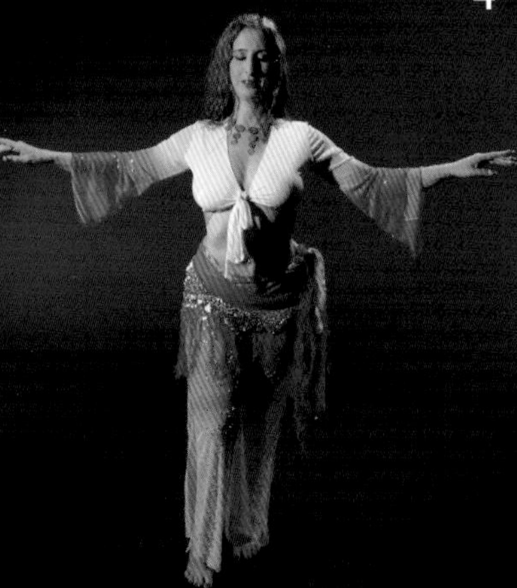

PRACTICE

Snap your hips sharply to the left and right for eight counts, then front and back for eight counts. Now try a belly dance technique called the "box" – this means sharply performing a dance step in four different directions: front, side, back and side. The hip snap box is based on four counts. Begin by snapping your hips to the left, then back, over to the right and finally to the front. Repeat four more times, then finish with two sets of side hip snaps.

HIP THRUST

1 Start in the foundation position (p.20), keeping your hips straight and knees softly bent. With your right foot, step about 60cm (2ft) to the right. Lift your heel, arching your foot, and place 70 percent of your weight on your supporting left leg.

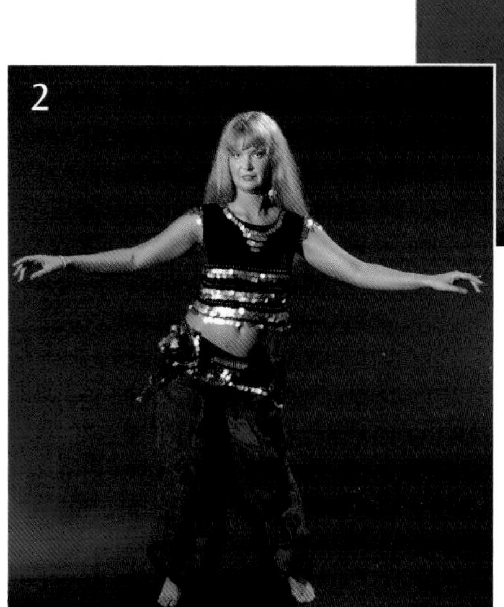

2 Isolating the rest of your body, thrust your right hip sharply up and out for one count. Slowly bring your hip back in, also for one count.

Pull your right leg back and step out with your left foot. Lift your left heel and thrust your hip out to the left for one count. Again, bring the hip back in for a single count.

Unlike the hip drops and lifts, the thrust is meant to be danced to two counts – one out, one in. You could speed it up to one count, but the music must be very fast for the step to look right.

HIP THRUST RETURN

A small adjustment to the hip thrust can add another dimension to the step. Starting again on the right side, instead of sharply thrusting your hips out, push them out gently and quickly snap them back into place. This accents the movement in instead of the movement out.

PRACTICE

Perform ten hip thrusts on your right side and ten on your left. Follow with alternate right and left hip thrusts.

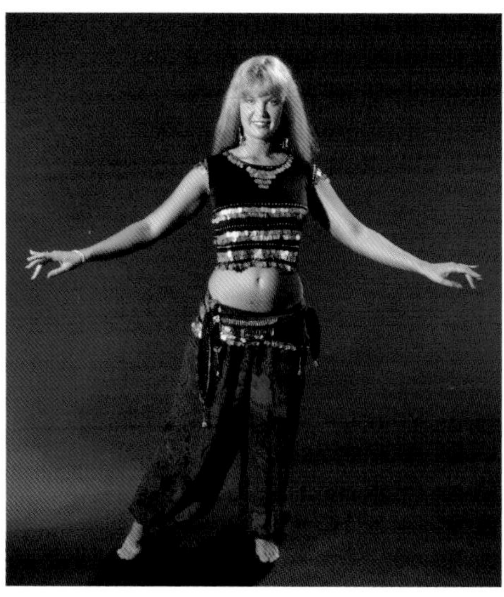

ADDING DETAIL

On the thrust, switch your hands into the offering position (p.21), then roll them back into basic (p.21) on the return.

JOINING THE HIP THRUST AND RETURN

Dance ten hip thrusts to each side, if possible without pausing in between. Follow with hip return thrusts on each side. Now, why not try accenting both the out and in movement?

HIP ROLLS

Although the hip roll movement draws attention to the hips, it is your footwork and leg strength that make it possible. The reverse hip roll is a more subtle movement – our anatomy prevents it being as broad and dramatic as the regular roll.

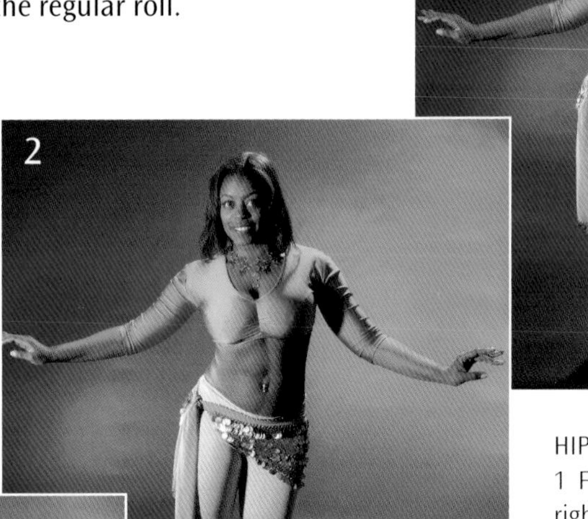

HIP ROLL

1 For the first count, step out to the right so that your feet are shoulder-width apart and flat on the ground. Sit out as far as you can to the right and bend your knees slightly. Your weight should be 70 percent on your right leg, 30 percent on your left.

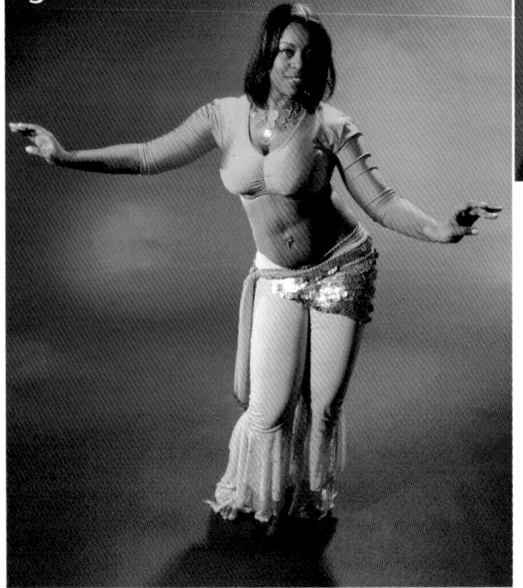

2 For the second count, arch your right foot as high as you can while tightly contracting the muscles that run down the right side of your torso. This will dramatically lift your hip. Make sure that you don't bob up and down by keeping your head and body at the same height as when you started the arch and contraction. Allowing your knees to bend and flex naturally with the hip roll helps you to keep level.

3 For the third count, roll your hips from the right to the left in one smooth movement. Push your hips as far as you can to the left, while shifting your weight to the left leg. Once you have rolled to the left, release your contracted muscles and drop your arched foot flat on the ground while sitting out. This final position is the perfect starting point for the left hip roll – repeat from step 1, but with your left hip.

PRACTICE

Practice and speed control will help you smooth out your hip rolls. Speed up the movements to two counts only and eliminate any pauses between steps. Try not to let your foot fall sharply to the floor, but place it down softly in a light release. After ten more two-count sets, speed up to only one count per roll. After ten of these, you should see the hip roll forming as you get used to the technique. At first it helps to repeat the following in your head while performing the rolls: right up, push, down, left up, push, down.

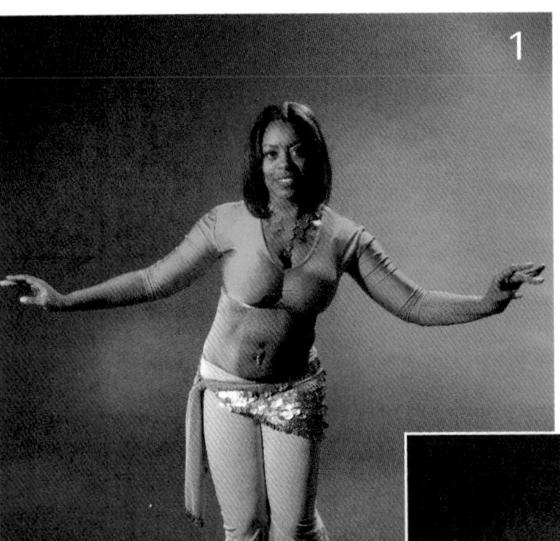

REVERSE HIP ROLL

1 Begin by moving into the beginning stance of a right hip roll, but don't push your hips so far. Remember to soften your knees and keep your height consistent.

2 Tightly contract the muscles on your left side and sharply arch your left foot. Unlike the hip roll in which you keep your hips thrust out while contracting, in the reverse hip roll you must keep your hip pulled in as close as possible to your center point during the lift and contraction.

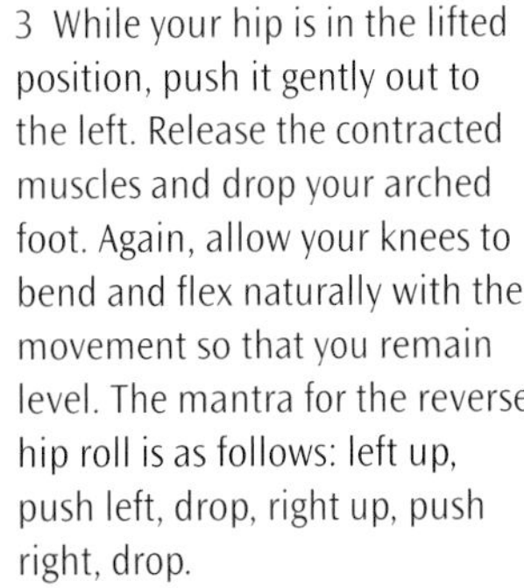

3 While your hip is in the lifted position, push it gently out to the left. Release the contracted muscles and drop your arched foot. Again, allow your knees to bend and flex naturally with the movement so that you remain level. The mantra for the reverse hip roll is as follows: left up, push left, drop, right up, push right, drop.

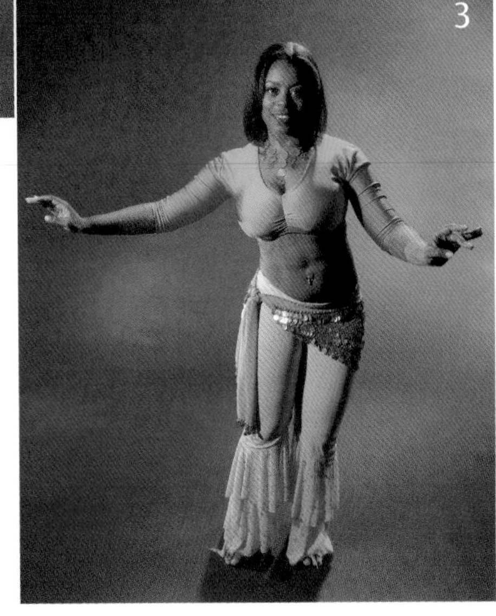

PRACTICE

Slowly repeat the reverse hip roll five times on each side. As with the regular hip roll, speed up to one count per roll and smooth it out.

To practice the hip roll and reverse hip roll together, first dance ten hip rolls, alternating left and right. Pause for one count and then move quickly into ten reverse hip rolls, alternating left and right.

VARIATION

During hip rolls and reverse hip rolls, try bending your knees deeply and dancing a few low rolls, gradually straightening your legs until you return to your normal height.

LARGE HIP CIRCLES

As with the hip rolls, the best way to learn the large hip circle is to break it down into four separate steps totalling eight counts, then bring the steps together.

PREPARATION

Stand in basic foundation (p.20), with your feet shoulder-width apart. As in the hip-releasing stretch (p.22), push your hips as far as you can to the right, keeping your feet flat on the floor, for two counts. Then push your hips to the left for two counts. Alternate between left and right for eight counts, then return to center.

Next, bend your knees about 7.5cm (3in) and contract your lower abdominal muscles. This will raise your pelvis and support your spine as you lean back slightly. Make sure that your lower back doesn't arch. Hold for two counts, then tilt your body forward until you have reversed your position.

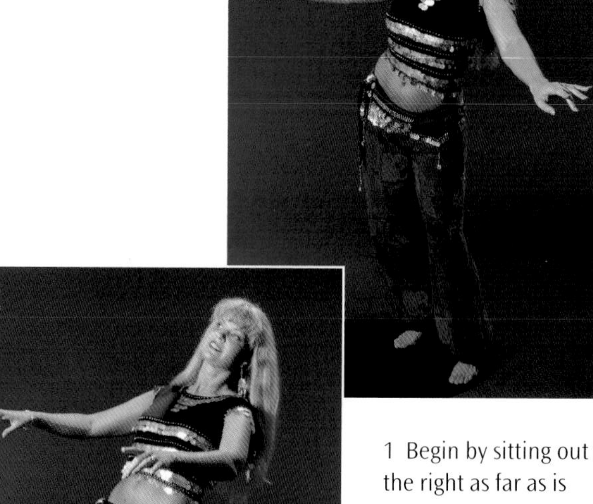

1 Begin by sitting out to the right as far as is comfortable for two counts.

2 Slowly round your hips forward, leaning back with your pelvis tucked under and your spine straight for two counts.

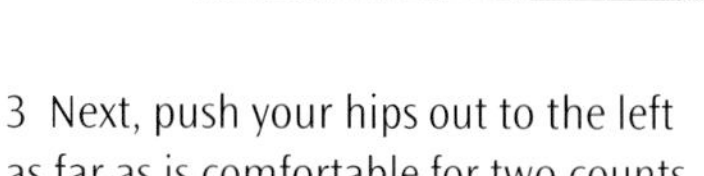

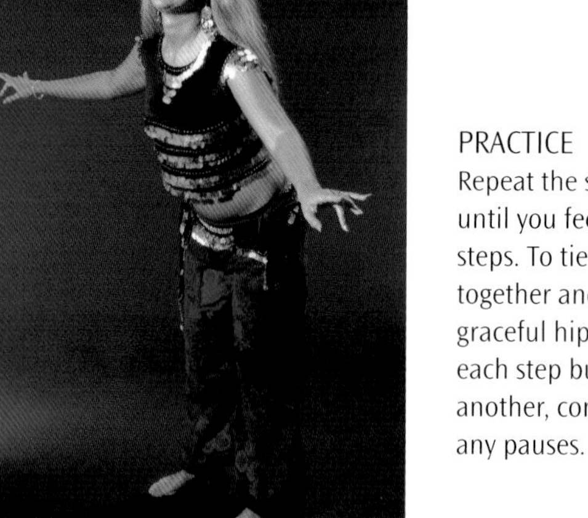

3 Next, push your hips out to the left as far as is comfortable for two counts.

4 Follow with a forward lean, again with a straight back, for two counts.

PRACTICE

Repeat the sequence four times until you feel confident with the steps. To tie the movements together and build a wide, graceful hip circle, don't hold each step but flow from one to another, connecting them without any pauses.

ADDING ELEGANT ARM MOVEMENTS

The addition of elegant arm movements will add visual interest and complexity to your hip circles.

1 For the first four counts as you round the circle to the right, switch your hands to the offering position (p.21).

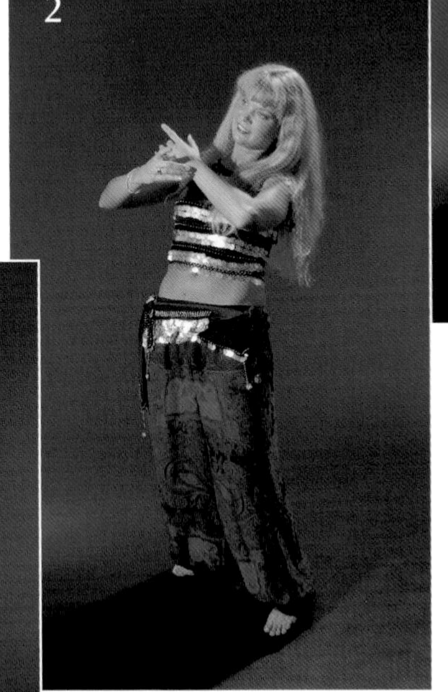

2, 3 Slowly bring your arms together at chest level, softly crossing them close to your body as your hips round from right to forward, back and left.

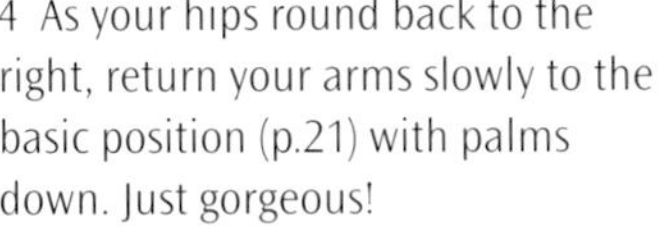

4 As your hips round back to the right, return your arms slowly to the basic position (p.21) with palms down. Just gorgeous!

PRACTICE

Perform four large hip circles with elegant arm movements to the right, followed by another four to the left. Experiment with changing the speed of the entire movement, alternating between left and right hip circles at fast and slow speeds.

HIP TWISTS

A fun, energetic movement, the hip twist can be danced on the spot or used as the hip twist walk, a travel step.

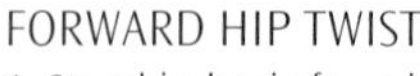

FORWARD HIP TWIST

1 Stand in basic foundation (p.20). On the first count, gently step forward on your left foot, planting it firmly on the ground in front of you.

2 Twist your left hip sharply forward and round to the right while turning your foot in the same direction. Softly twist your hip back to the starting position while gently lifting your foot off the floor in a small kick. Put your foot back down in the same place you kicked off from and dance another hip twist. Repeat eight times, then switch to the right hip.

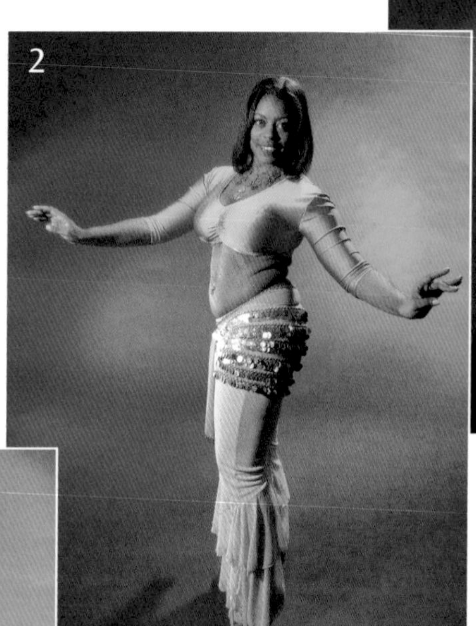

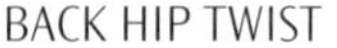

BACK HIP TWIST

3 Begin by performing a forward hip twist, but do not forcefully thrust your hip forward. Just softly extend it with a gentle push.

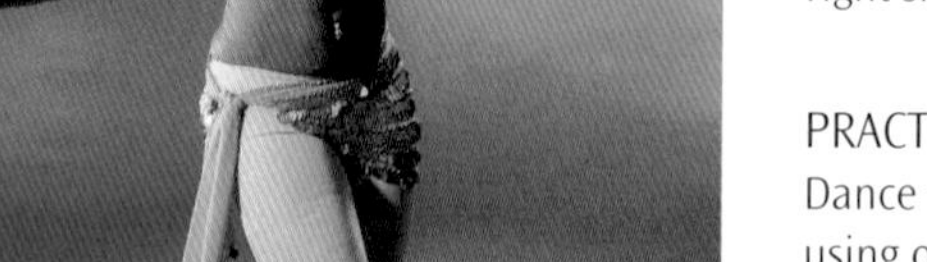

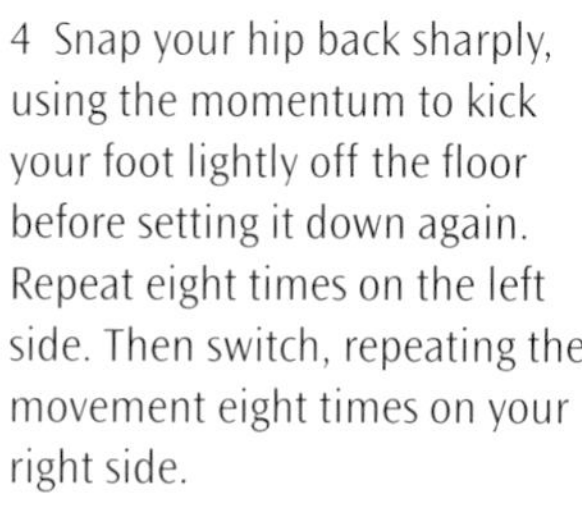

4 Snap your hip back sharply, using the momentum to kick your foot lightly off the floor before setting it down again. Repeat eight times on the left side. Then switch, repeating the movement eight times on your right side.

PRACTICE

Dance the forward hip twist using one count for each step. Twist on the left for eight counts (four twists), then speed up until only one beat is required for a full twist. Repeat on the right side. Follow with a full set of back hip twists on both sides with the same tempo as above.

HIP TWIST WALK

1 Perform a full left hip twist, accentuating the forward motion.

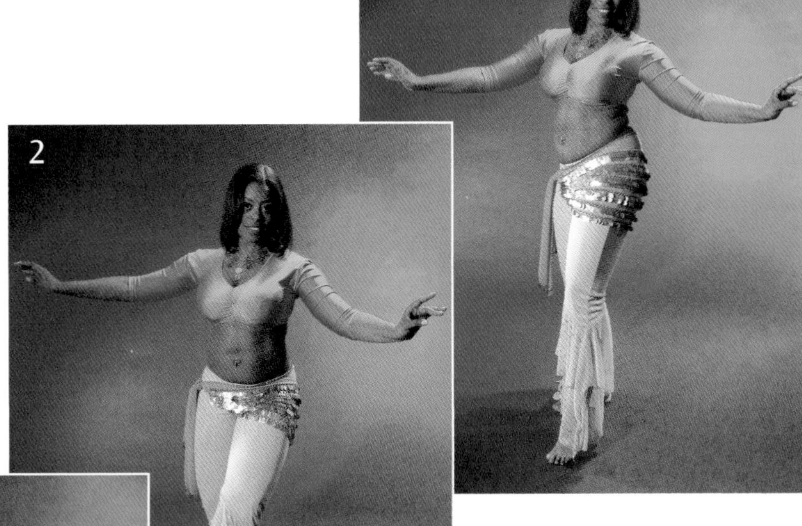

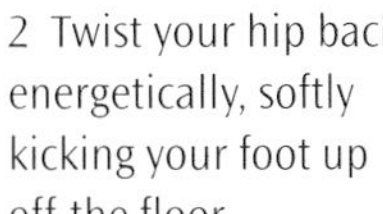

2 Twist your hip back energetically, softly kicking your foot up off the floor.

3 Instead of placing your left foot back down for another hip twist, use it to take a large step, about 30cm (12in), forward, turning your toes moderately out to the left.

4 Immediately step forward with your right foot, moving quickly into a right hip twist. As your right foot lifts off the ground, take a large step forward. Now quickly step forward with your left foot, repeating the entire segment from the beginning. Continue alternating left and right. This easy travel step will take you right across the floor if you let it!

VARIATION

Feel free to dance as many hip twists as you like between each walk step.

THE BODY INTENSE SHIMMY

The body intense shimmy demonstrates belly dancing's roots in fertility and the ritualistic act of giving birth better than any other movement. It's also the most widely recognized step and unique to belly dance.

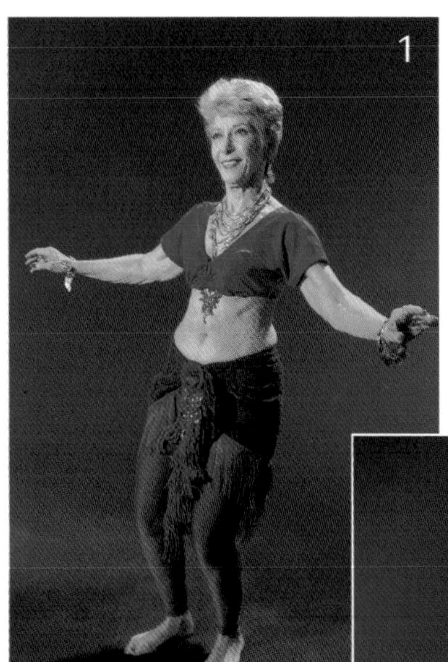

1 Contrary to popular belief, the shimmy emanates from the knees, not the hips! Select some music with a rapid tempo and stand in foundation (p.20). Modify your foundation pose by placing your feet side by side and flat on the ground. Relax your knees, bending them slightly so that they are loose and supple.

Take a few long breaths. Many of us have a tendency to hold our breath and contract our muscles when doing something strenuous, such as shimmying, but that is the fastest way to run out of energy. As you learn to shimmy, breathing evenly and deeply will help you keep going longer and prevent your knees from locking.

2 Bend your right knee and notice that your left hip lifts slightly. Do not lock your left knee and try your best to keep it soft. Return your right knee to its starting position, also without straightening or locking it.

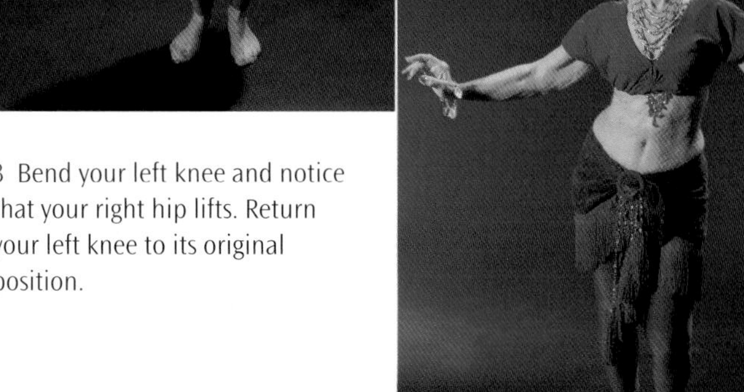

3 Bend your left knee and notice that your right hip lifts. Return your left knee to its original position.

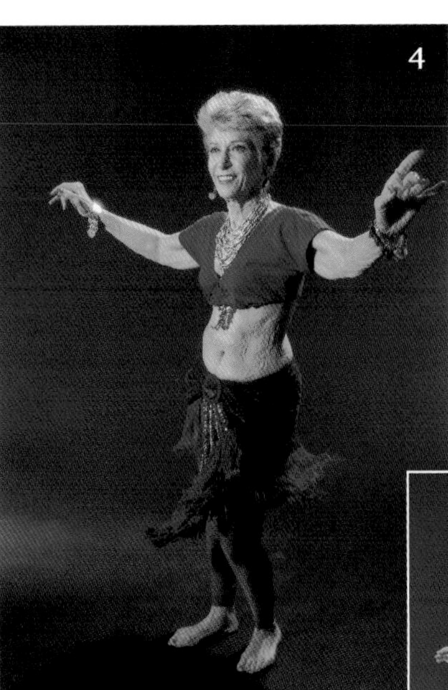

4 Now slowly bend your knees, alternating left and right. As each knee rises and drops so will the opposite hip. This is the cornerstone of the shimmy. Remember not to straighten your legs so much that your knees lock. Keep them soft.

Gradually speed up your knee bends until you feel you can go no faster. There you are – that is a fully fledged shimmy!

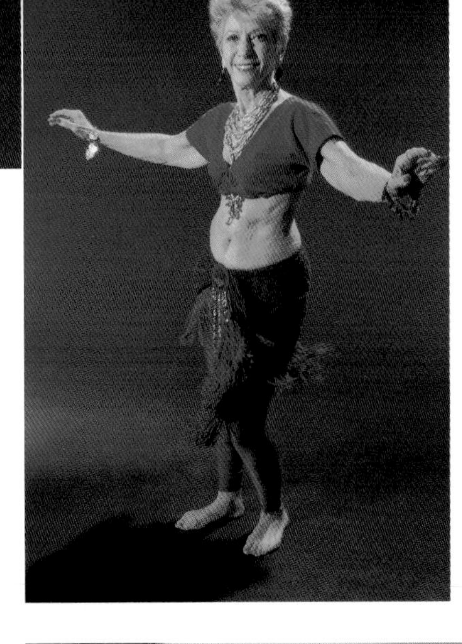

5 After about a minute or so of shimmying, you may start to feel a burn in your thigh muscles – that means you are doing the movement properly. After two minutes of shimmying, you may start to sweat and that's even better. Shimmying takes incredible energy, so sweating is another sign that you are moving the correct way. Once the shimmy motor is running, you can relax and your body will almost shimmy by itself.

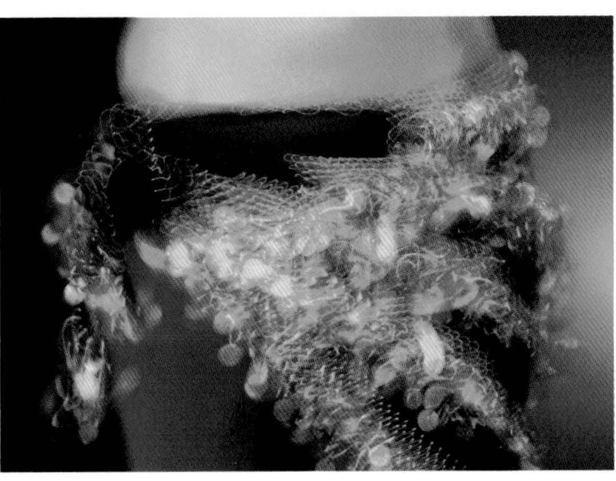

SHAKE THAT BELT

A coin belt is a wonderful prop when learning to shimmy. The spirited sound not only serves as an inspiration but also indicates the speed of your shimmy.

BELLY ROLL

Don't be disheartened if you aren't able to perform this movement straight away. It takes time to develop the muscle control necessary to roll your entire abdomen. Keep trying and you will get there.

PREPARATION
Place your hands on your belly, one above the other. Fully relax your stomach – let it hang as though it has no muscles at all. Take a deep breath in and then breathe out, feeling the muscles under your hands working. The lower abdomen is generally engaged before the upper abdomen. Repeat three more times until you are in tune with your breathing.

Relax your stomach again and, rather than waiting for a breath, contract ONLY your lower abdominal muscles. Relax. Then contract ONLY your upper ab muscles. Now that you have an idea of the different muscles, try a belly roll.

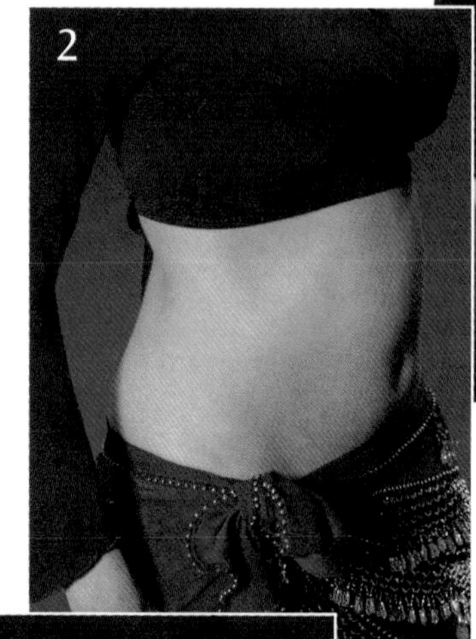

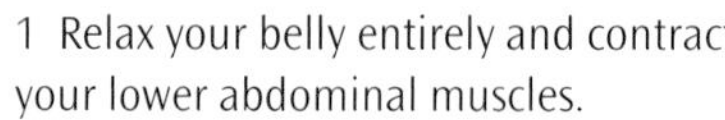

1 Relax your belly entirely and contract your lower abdominal muscles.

2 Gradually release the lower abs and simultaneously begin to contract the upper ones.

3 As your upper abs clench and pull in close to your body, fully relax your lower abs.

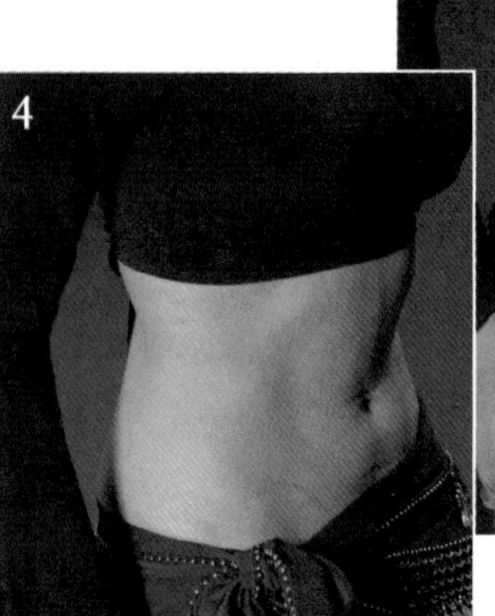

4 Finally, flex your lower abs while relaxing the upper muscles, then begin the series again. If you can do this four or five times successfully you will find yourself performing a bona fide belly roll as you contract and release your abdominal muscles.

VARIATION
Once you can do the normal belly roll, try it in reverse! Instead of starting by contracting the lower abdominal muscles, contract the upper ones, then move on to the lower. As you contract the lower set, release the upper abdominals so that the roll appears to reverse direction and wave down rather than up.

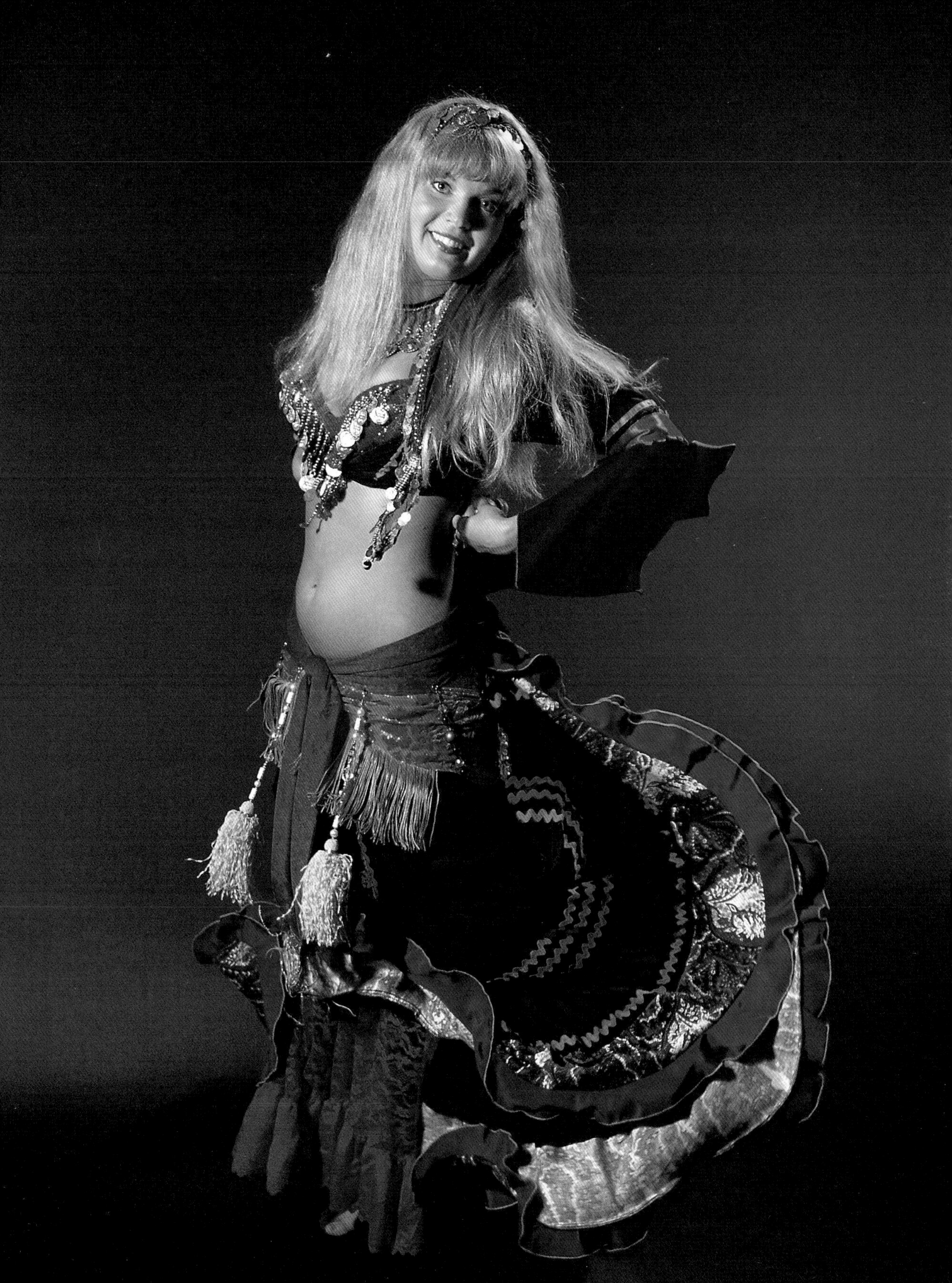

SENSUOUS UNDULATION

Another staple in belly dance, the undulation is both unusual and sensual without being overtly suggestive. Pulling the undulation sequence together takes patience and practice. It is especially important that you look in a mirror as you try this technique so that you can see your entire body working and make sure you're moving correctly.

PREPARATION STEPS FOR UNDULATION

Instead of facing front in the foundation stance, turn your body until you are at a 45-degree angle to the mirror. Thrust your chest forward as far as you can for two counts, arching your upper spine and pushing your shoulders back (see chest thrust p.44). Then roll your shoulders forward and compress your upper body into a deep slouch for two counts. Repeat both the thrust and the slouch four more times.

Now, using parts of the hip circle (p.34), tuck your pelvis up by contracting your abdominal muscles and lean back with bent knees for two counts. Lift up from your chest while straightening your knees moderately and lean forward, hinging at the waist, also for two counts. Repeat four times.

PUTTING THE MOVEMENT TOGETHER

In order to develop the necessary clean, snakelike movements, you now need to connect the four two-count steps detailed above into an eight-count undulation. Remember, taking it slowly and speeding up gradually is the best way to develop muscle control and learn this technique correctly.

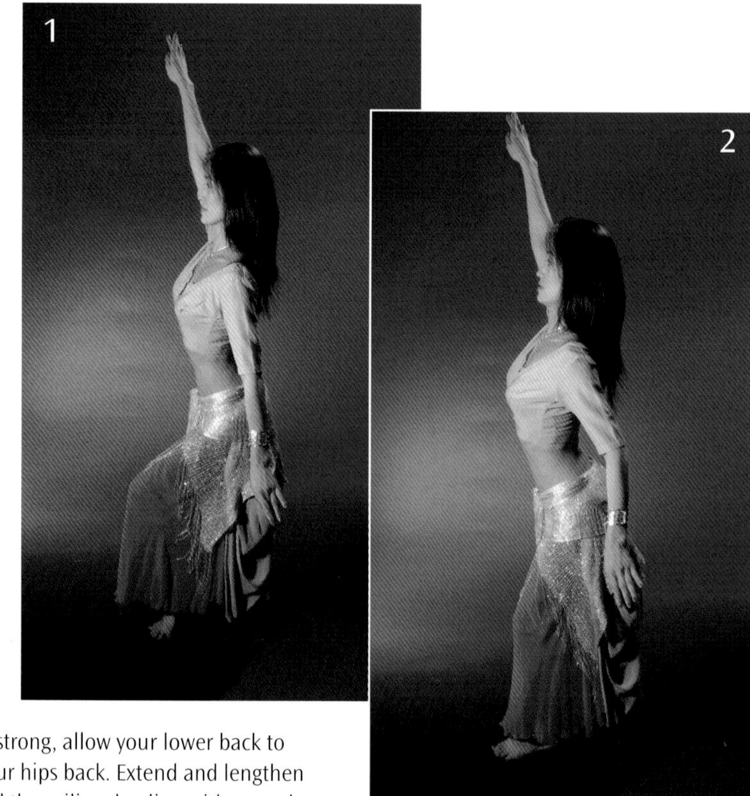

1 Begin with the arch. Firmly push your chest as far forward as you can, keeping your shoulders pressed back.

2 Keeping the arch strong, allow your lower back to release and push your hips back. Extend and lengthen your body up toward the ceiling, leading with your chest.

3 Start to lean back. Support your lower spine by tucking your pelvis slightly up and in.

4 With knees softly bent, continue to lean back as far as you can go without any strain to your spine or abdominal muscles.

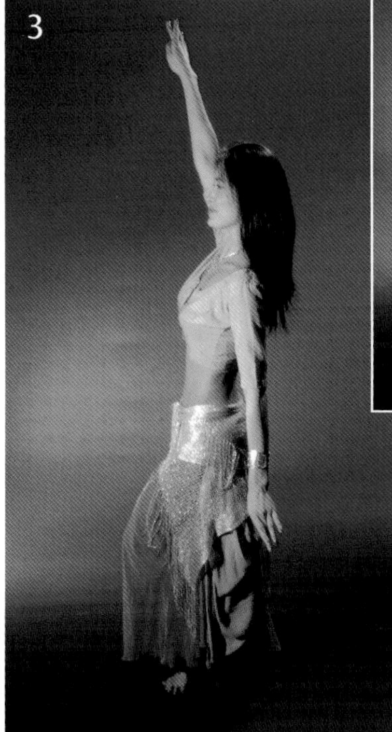

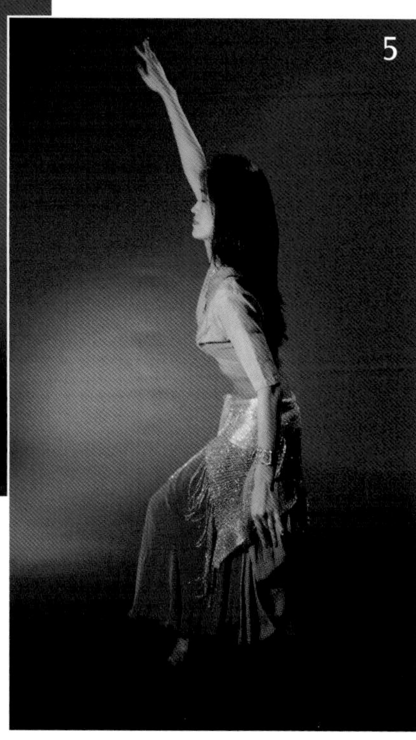

5 Curl in your chest and roll your upper body forward until your entire body is almost crouched into a reverse C shape.

To finish the undulation, strongly arch your chest out and push your hips back again. Continue with the forward momentum and lead with your chest until you rise up and slide into the beginning position. Keep repeating the undulation with as few pauses as possible. It will be choppy in the beginning, but as your body grows accustomed to the movements, it will smooth out.

PRACTICE

Dance four undulations with your body facing 45 degrees to the right, then four more with your body entirely in profile. Switch to the left profile and dance four undulations, then turn 45 degrees to the left and dance four more. As you grow accustomed to moving your body in this way, try to avoid the tendency to speed up. An undulation is meant to be slow and soothing like ocean waves, not wiggly like a worm. Only when you are sure that you've mastered the movement should you consider adding speed as a variation.

VARIATION: HIGH/LOW UNDULATIONS

Standing in foundation (p.20), step forward on your right foot in a rocking motion. Then rock back on your left foot. Practice this gentle sway for 16 counts, two counts forward and two counts back. When the next forward rock begins, arch your chest forward and begin the undulation. As you rock back, finish the undulation with the lower part of your body.

Try adding a dip to the undulation by bending your knees on one full undulating rock back and forth, then standing on your toes for a second full rock back and forth. Alternate between high and low undulations while rocking on your feet for a count of 16.

CHEST THRUSTS AND CHEST CIRCLES

CHEST THRUST SIDE TO SIDE

1 Keeping your shoulders relaxed and your hips directly over your legs, isolate your chest and thrust it out to the right as far as you can. Imagine that your legs and hips are frozen solid and there is a rope around your shoulders pulling you directly to the right.

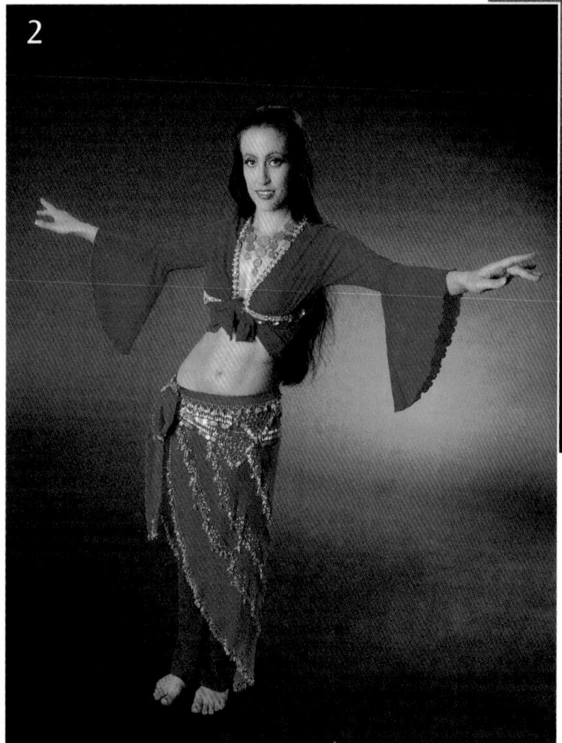

2 Return to the center and push to the left. The visual effect should be that the upper and lower halves of your body are on two separate planes and are moving independently of one another.

If it looks as if you are not really moving, but simply bending your chest to the left and right in almost a slump on each side, try counteracting this by slightly lifting the shoulder on the side in which you are thrusting. In other words, if you are pushing your chest to the right, lightly lift your right shoulder. When you are pushing to the left, gently lift your left shoulder. This will square out the upper part of your body, making the movement distinct.

PRACTICE

Perform ten chest thrusts, alternating to the left and right, for two counts each. Then speed up to one count on each side. Try playing with the timing by holding a left thrust for two counts, then alternating right and left for one count and vice versa.

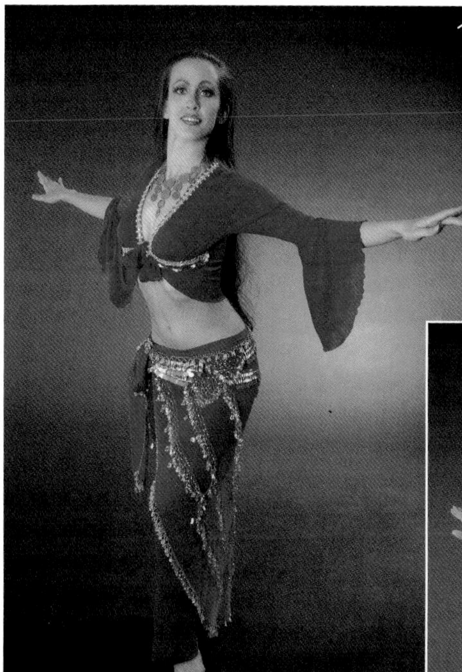

CHEST THRUST FRONT AND BACK

1 Chest thrusts can be danced front to back as well as side to side. Imagine that instead of pulling you right and left, the rope is now pulling you forward and back. Thrust your chest forward as far as you can, pulling your shoulders back and arching your upper spine.

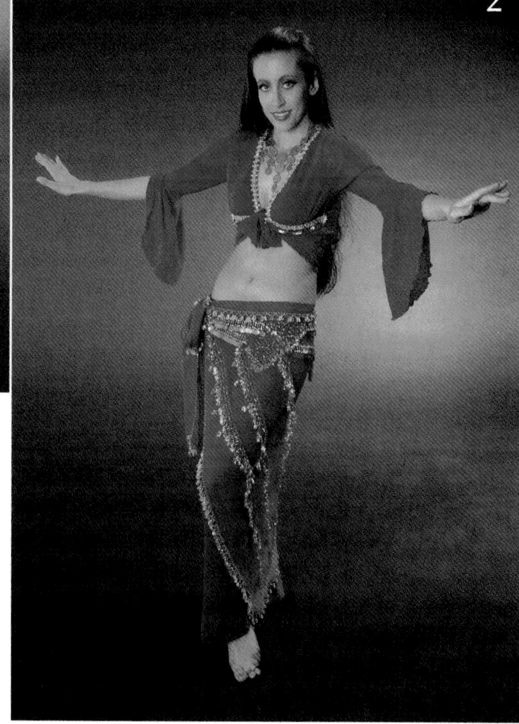

2 Then roll your shoulders forward and curve your back so that it appears as if you are slouching, with your chest caving in.

CHEST CIRCLES

Perform a "box" (p.30) of chest thrusts with your upper body. Each move should be two counts. Thrust forward, return to center. Push to the right, return to center. Thrust back, return to center. Push to the left, return to center. Next, repeat the box, but without returning to center after each movement. Repeat five times, then smooth the sequence out. Remove any pauses in between steps and slowly rotate your chest to each point using one count. A chest circle will take a total of four counts to achieve.

CHEST THRUST PRACTICE

Alternate between pushing forward and back ten times for two counts each. Try experimenting with timing as you did with the side to side thrusts.

CHEST CIRCLE PRACTICE

Perform a chest circle for four more four-count rotations, then speed up to two-count rotations in each direction.

BEAUTIFUL BACKBENDS

This step should be learned gradually. Only increase the arch when your back is fully supported by strong, well-developed abdominal and lower back muscles.

WARNING
If you have, or have had, any spinal or neck pain or injury, do not perform this movement under any circumstances. Even if you are without pain or injury, try this step only with the aid of another person, who can catch you if you start to fall over backwards.

1 Stand with your feet shoulder-width apart and your hands in basic one (p.21). On your dominant side, step directly back with the corresponding foot. Step far enough to bring the toes of your back foot in line with the heel of your front foot. Unlock your knees and allow them to bend softly.

Contract your abdominals and tuck your pelvis slightly forward. Keeping your abdominal muscles tight will support and straighten your lower back. It is very important not to allow your lower spine to collapse onto itself so keep those abs rock solid!

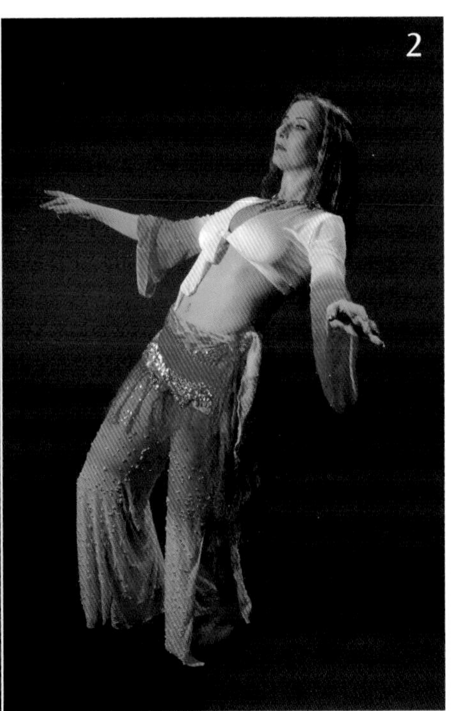
2

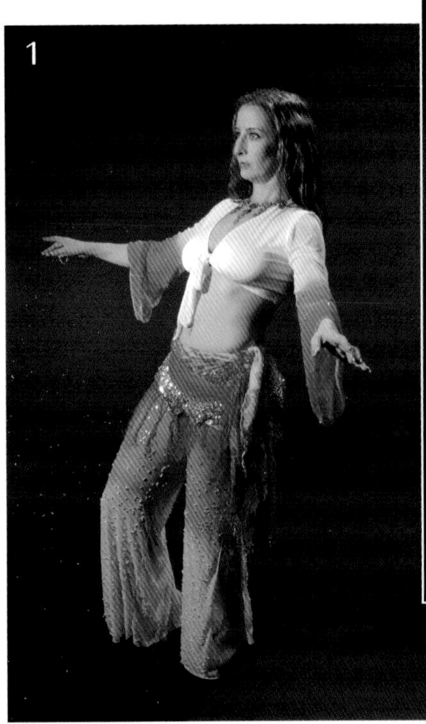
1

2 Tilt your head back slightly and, keeping your shoulders pressed down, slowly bend back about 7.5cm (3in). Allow your knees to bend naturally with the movement. Pause and check your body to make sure your lower back isn't arching yet. If this is easy for you, go back another 7.5cm (3in). Check your body again. If you are feeling strain in your neck or spine, slowly come up again. This means that your muscles are not developed enough to go farther and you must only drop this far until they are strong enough to do more.

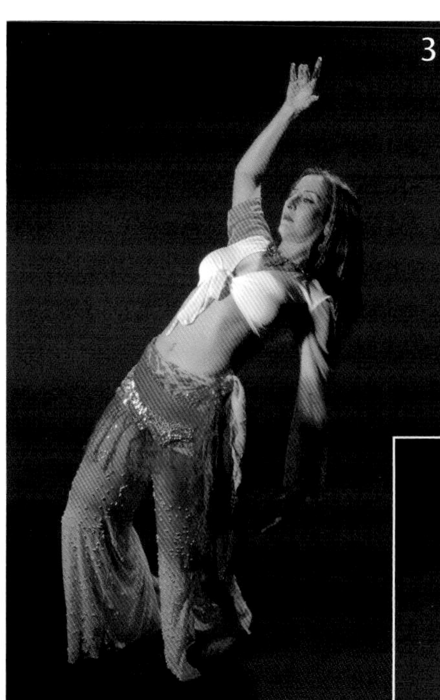

3 If you still feel comfortable, drop back another 7.5cm (3in) and raise the arm opposite your supporting leg.

4 Continue to dip back slowly by 7.5cm (3in) increments until the first sign of strain, then come back up 7.5cm (3in). This point is your maximum range until your muscles are stronger.

If your neck and upper back feel very strong, gently tilt your head back and look at the ceiling. Hold for a few moments. Slowly come back up, leading with your chest.

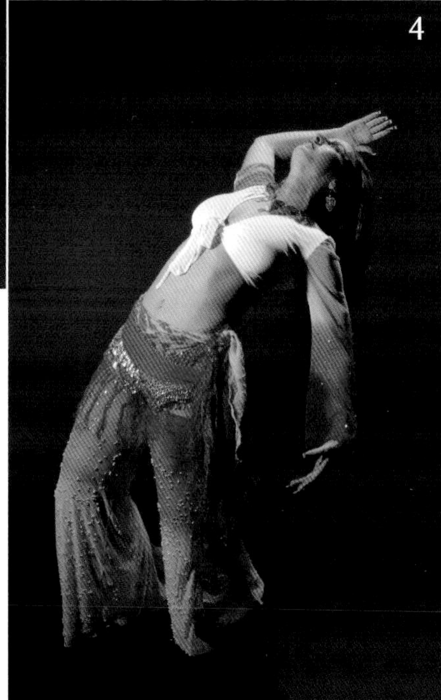

PRACTICE

As you fall gently into your backbend, note at which point you start to develop tension in your neck and spine and come back up. Fall back again, this time holding the backbend at the very point before you feel the strain for five seconds. Repeat five times. Break for a minute or two, then repeat. If you practice every day, your backbend should become deeper and more secure as your muscles gain strength.

ADDING ELEGANT ARM MOVEMENTS

Making the backbend beautiful is easier than the backbend itself. Raise your arms in front of you and simply strike a pretty pose with your hands. Use basic hands or offering hands (p.21) to make this technique look more elegant and less gymnastic. Adding forward snake arms (p.54) is another wonderful way to enhance the movement without drawing attention away from the bend itself.

COBRA NECK SLITHER

Begin by repeating the neck stretches (p.22) before attempting the cobra neck slither. The unusual head movements in belly dance are unlike anything in Western dance styles.

PREPARATION

Inhale deeply and relax your shoulders. Place your fingertips on your neck, directly below the angle of your jawbone. Gently circle your fingers until you find the muscle underneath. This is the muscle you need to engage to perform the cobra. Gently slide your neck to the right. As you do, feel the muscle on the left side of your neck moving. Repeat in the other direction, feeling the muscles on the right side work. This movement is more of a push than a pull, so it is important not to overextend your neck. Even just a small movement in each direction is enough to make an impact. As your neck becomes more flexible from doing neck stretches and the slither, your range will improve.

1 Raise your arms up above your head so they are parallel to your ears. Firmly press your shoulders down and back, un-crowding your neck. Place your palms together and lower them until your elbows are bent at a 45-degree angle. This lovely face frame is a perfect complement to the cobra.

2, 3 Now, as you practiced, simply slither your head left, then right. Make sure you don't tilt your head in the direction you are moving to compensate for limited neck flexibility. It's best to perform the movement correctly, no matter how small. To add a further oriental touch, smile a little and move your eyes back and forth in the direction of your slither.

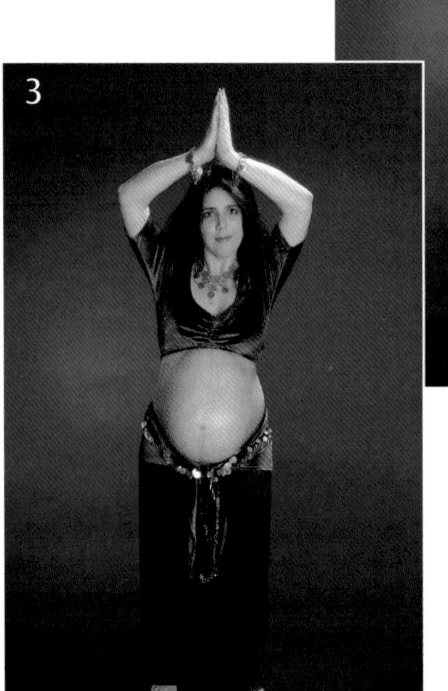

VARIATION

Instead of standing still and placing your palms together with straight wrists, twist your wrists and cross them, meeting the palms in the middle (right). Step dramatically forward, slithering as you go.

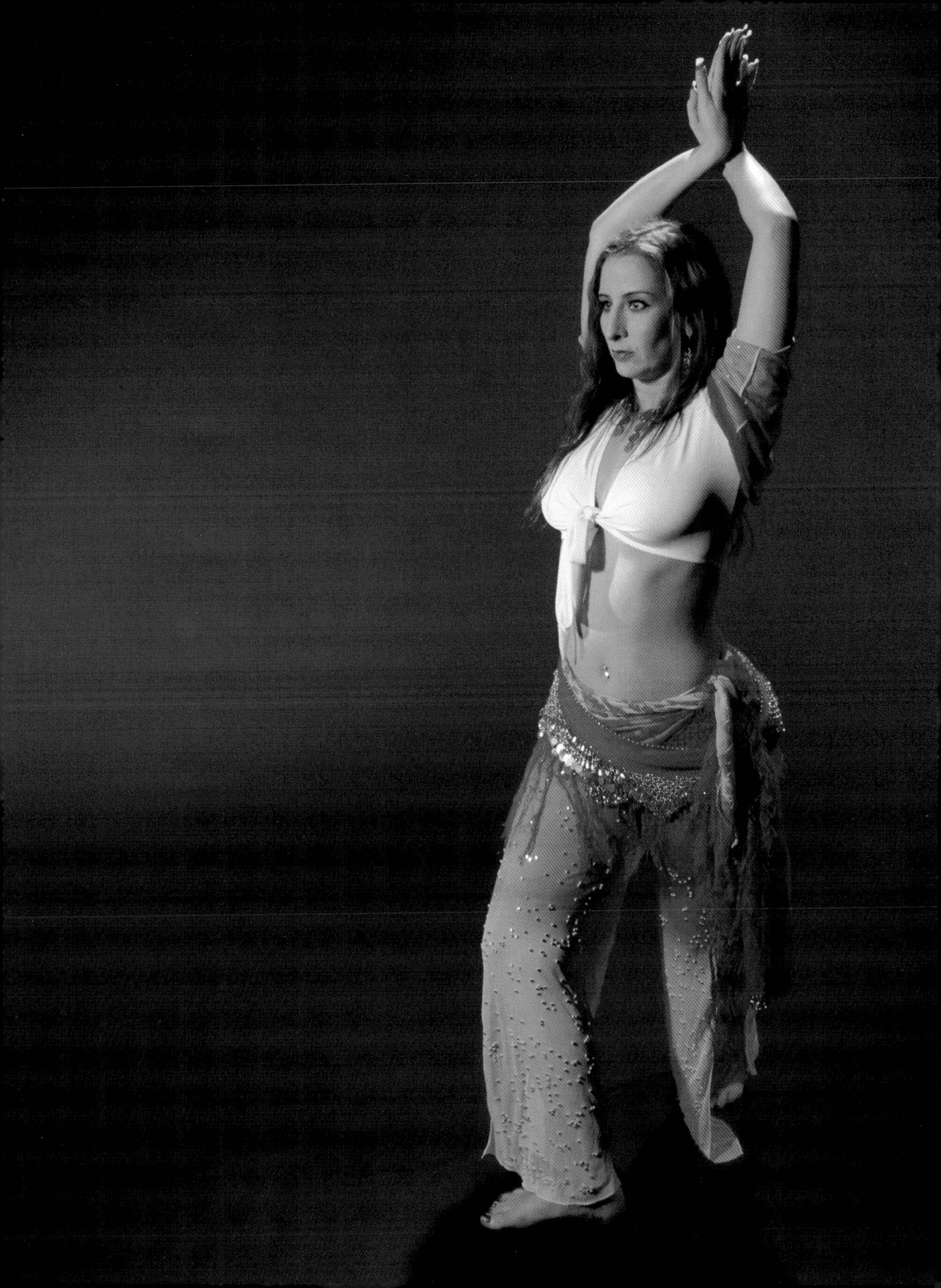

POSES

Here are some examples of beautiful hand and arm poses you can use in your dance. Posing during a dance routine is an excellent way for the dancer to have a short break, while allowing observers to take in visual details that might otherwise be missed.

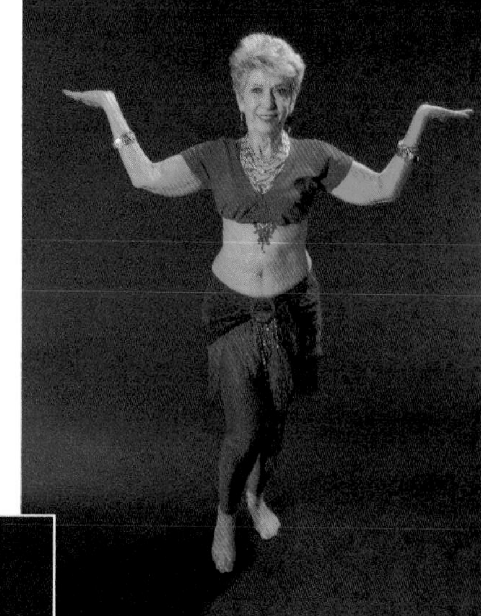

OFFERING

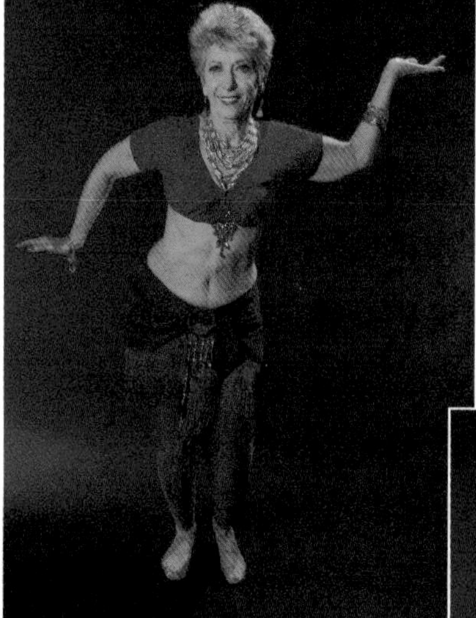

ARABY PUSH

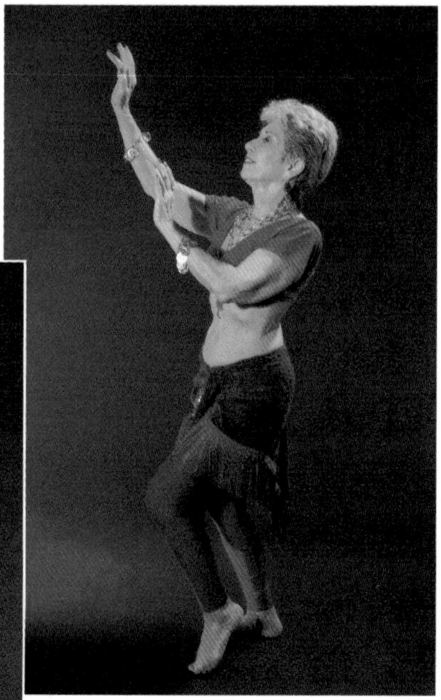

EGYPTIAN GODDESS

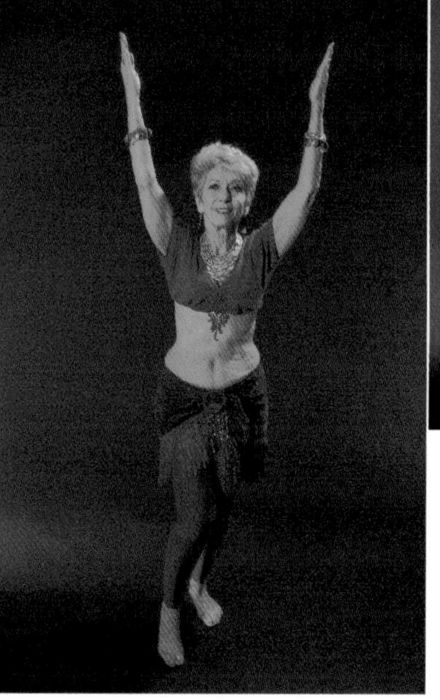

FINALE POSTURE: RA'S CROWN

SHOULDER SHAKE

Use your shoulders to express a wide range of feelings and concepts in belly dancing. Just as you can say "I don't know" by shrugging your shoulders, you can also express flirtation, playfulness – even pride – by shoulder movements as you dance.

1 Stand in foundation with basic arms (p.20). Look at the position of your hands and imagine that each one is resting on a wall so that it cannot move. Relax your shoulders completely and raise them about 1cm (½in) or so.

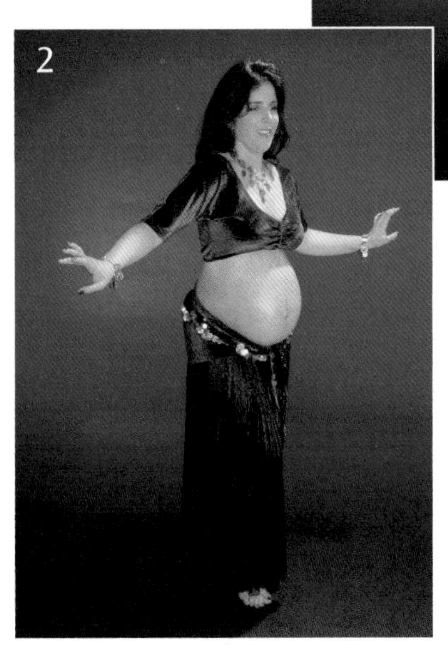

2 Push your right shoulder forward without moving your arm or hand – remember, there is a wall there. Repeat eight times, making sure you keep your arm still. Perform another set, but now sharpen the movement by putting the accent on the push. Switch to your left shoulder and repeat for eight counts on the left side. Again, repeat and sharpen the movement for eight counts. Alternate your shoulders left and right sharply, so as one shoulder is pushed out, the other is pulled in.

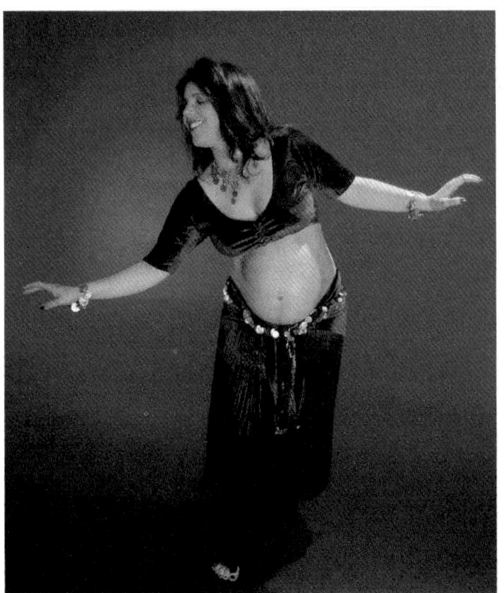

VARIATION

For a playful, 1930s-style belly dance step, dip your body slowly to the left, center, then right, while practicing the shoulder shake. This is a classic belly dance movement which, when combined with the shoulder shake, takes you right back to the sultan's palace!

PRACTICE

Alternate pushing each shoulder forward for two counts, totalling 16 beats. Speed up to one count per push and soften the movement so it becomes a gentle shake, rather than sharp accents. Don't overdo the shake – the focus is meant to be on your shoulders, not other parts of you!

HAND MOVEMENTS

These movements are often the last skills to be mastered by a new belly dancer. The need for grace and subtlety means that hands must be used conservatively, so as not to draw attention away from other parts of the body. You may find that these beautiful positions carry over into your everyday life – in the way you hold a teacup, use your hands as you speak, or even in the way you rest your hands at a computer keyboard.

CIRCLING HANDS

Practice this simple technique of circling hands from basic one (p.21) to basic two, or offering hand (p.21), every day until it becomes second nature. It will make a wonderful difference in your dancing and can be used in just about any of the dance steps.

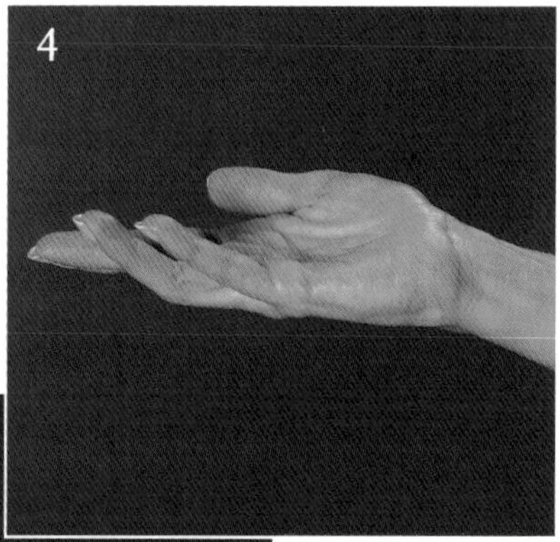

4

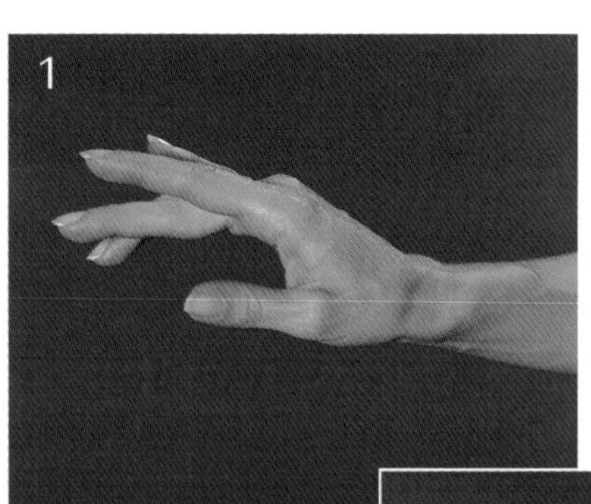

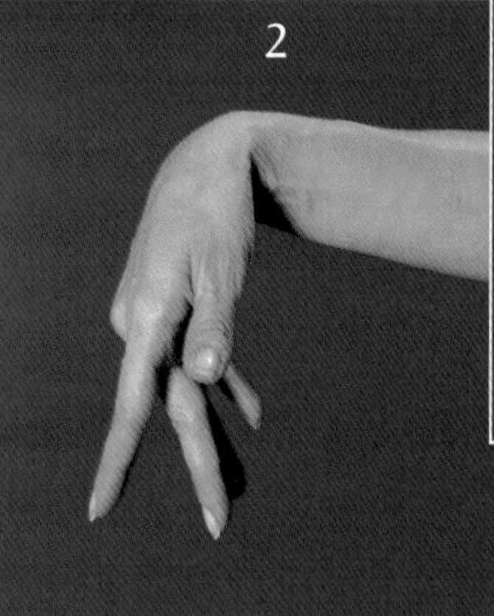

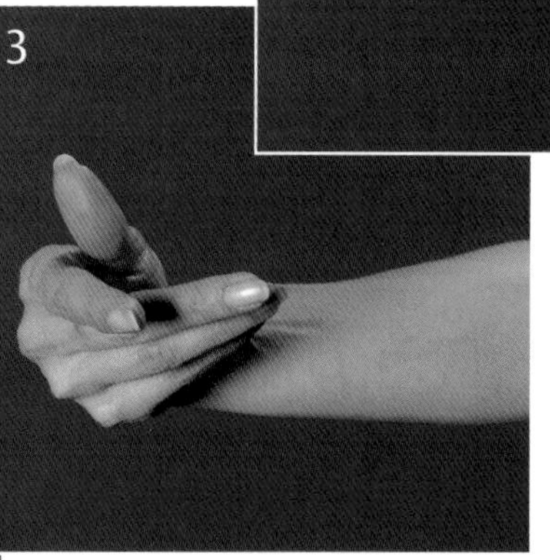

1 Start with your right hand in basic one position.

2 Drop your wrist and stiffen your fingers while sweeping your hand counterclockwise in a full half circle.

3 Continue to rotate your wrist until your forearm and palm are facing up.

4 Release your stiffened fingers into basic two, or the offering hand position.

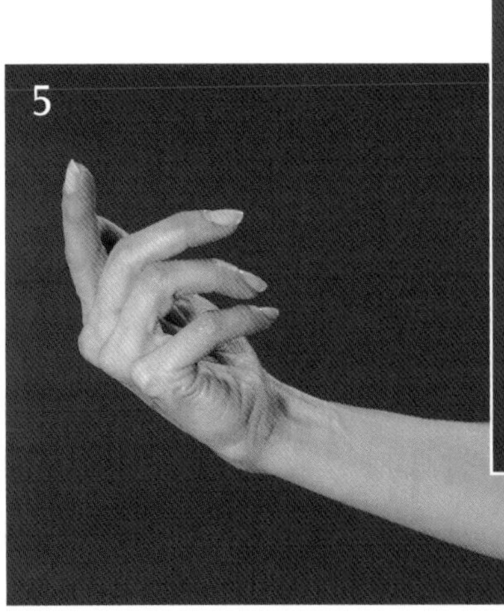

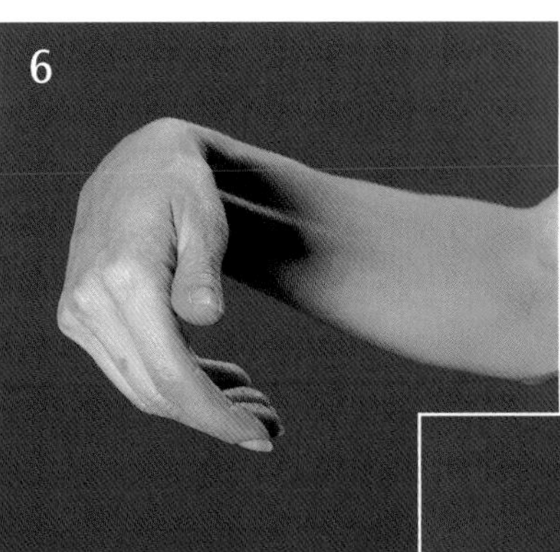

5 Straighten your wrist and, gently curling your fingers, softly fold your hand at the base knuckles.

6 Rotate your wrist clockwise while sweeping your hand down and around until the palm and forearm are facing down.

7 Then, smoothly drop your wrist while lifting your hand, returning your fingers to basic one.

SPANISH HANDS

When the Arabs inhabited Spain, the cultures had an interesting impact on each other. You can see the cross-cultural influence in this Spanish hands technique. A powerful modification on circling hands, it adds further elegance to those simple movements.

1 Start by holding one hand, bent at the wrist in basic one position (p.21), over your head, with fingers pointing at the ceiling. The other hand should also be in basic one, but held at waist level, fingers pointing down. Starting with the index fingers on the upper and lower hands, fold over each finger at the base knuckles one at a time, while rotating your wrists around in a circle (see basic to offering hand switch, opposite).

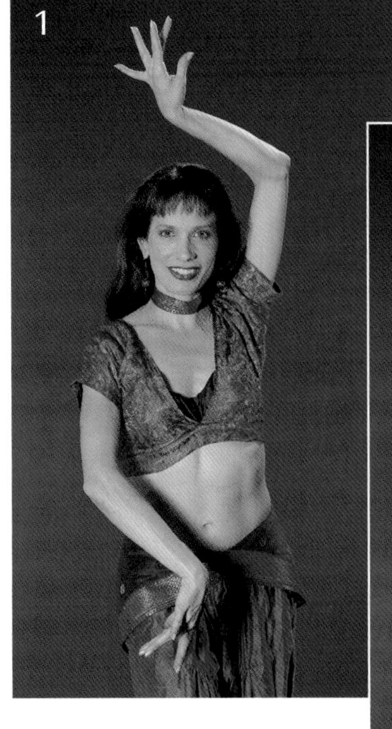

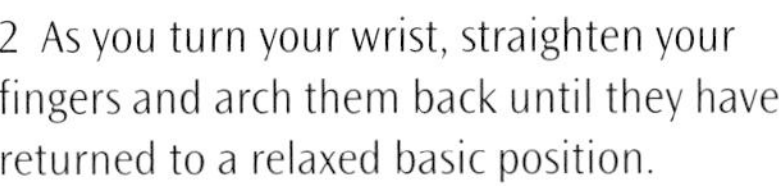

2 As you turn your wrist, straighten your fingers and arch them back until they have returned to a relaxed basic position.

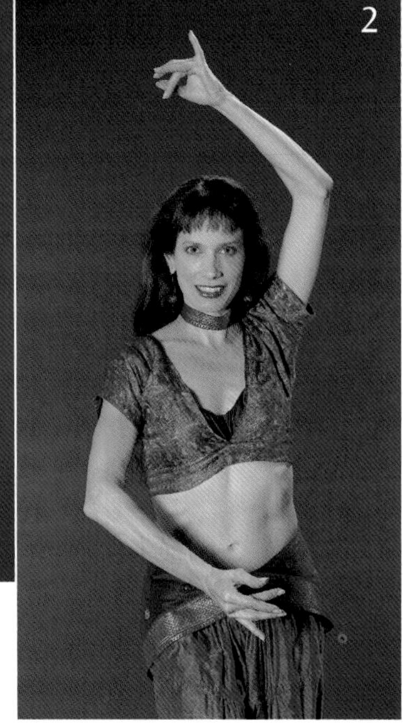

SNAKE ARMS

Sensuous and almost eerie, snake arms are meant to entice and hypnotize. Start by learning the single snake arms, then move on to the alternating version.

SINGLE SNAKE ARMS

1 Stand with your feet flat on the floor and arms at your sides, palms facing inward. Lift your right arm, keeping it slightly bent at the elbow as if holding a large rolled-up towel under your arm. Roll your shoulder forward so that your elbow is pointing toward the ceiling.

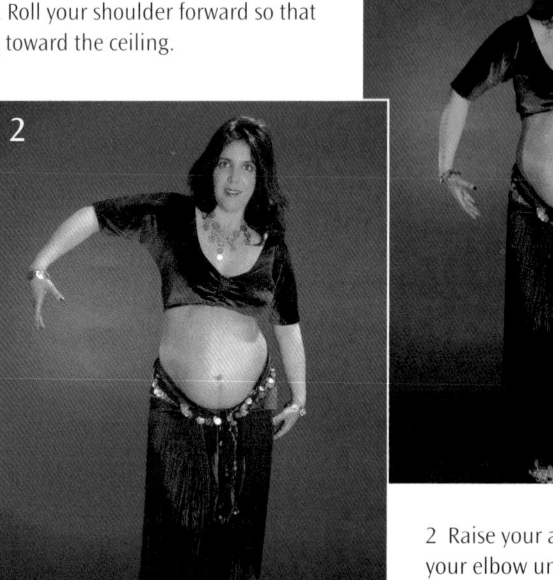

2 Raise your arm, leading with your elbow until it is just above shoulder height, or as high as you can manage. Beginning with your wrist, lift your hand gradually.

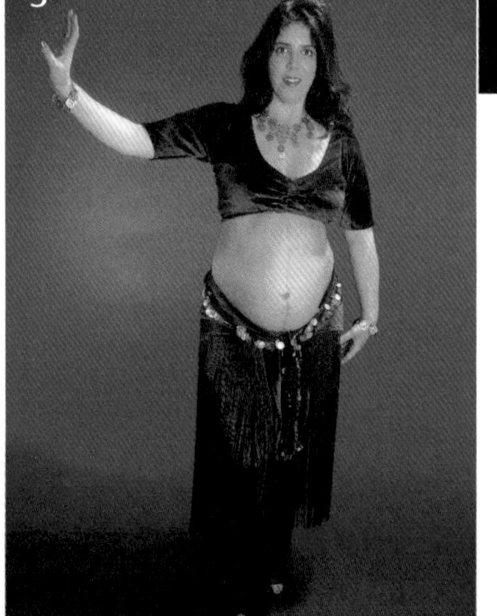

3 As your hand continues to lift, rotate your elbow to point down. Softly bend your fingers and turn your palm out, while gradually lowering your arm until it is at your side. Repeat the step eight times, then start again with your left arm.

DON'T WORRY!

The muscles used to perform these techniques are rarely used in daily life. Don't be surprised if you find that after practicing this movement your arms and hands are shaky. This is a natural result of tired muscles and will pass in a few hours.

ALTERNATING SNAKE ARMS

1 Begin with your right arm, slowly lifting it until you rotate your elbow and change the direction of your hand. At the moment when you begin to drop your right arm, start the step on the left side of your body by raising your left arm.

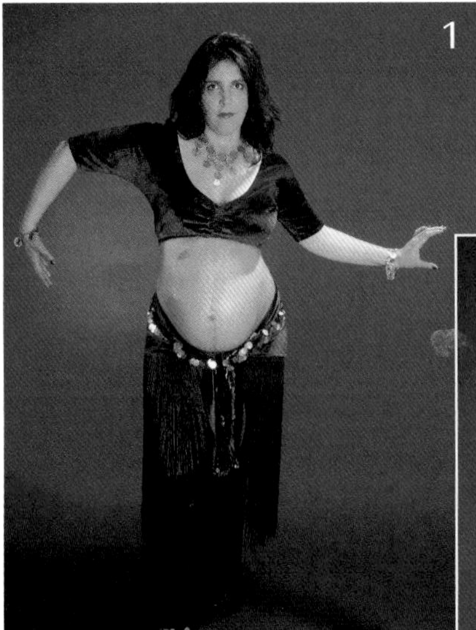

2 As your left elbow reaches shoulder level and rotates to turn down, your right arm should be once again beginning its ascent. Each arm should be working slowly in the opposite direction to the other. This technique takes lots of coordination so be patient and take it slowly.

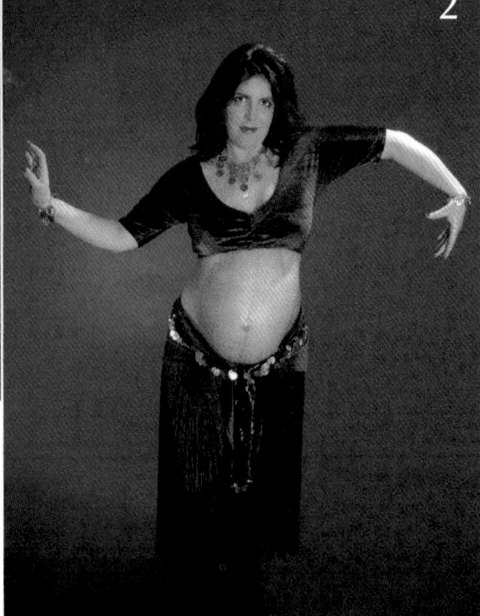

PRACTICE

Begin by snaking both arms at the same time for four counts as you raise them, and four counts as you lower them. Then lift only the left for four counts, followed by the right for four counts. Move back into snaking both arms together. Finally, as the arms come back down, lift only the left. As you begin to lower it, immediately bring up the right to start alternating snake arms. Speed up the alternating snake arms to two counts per movement. Repeat six times.

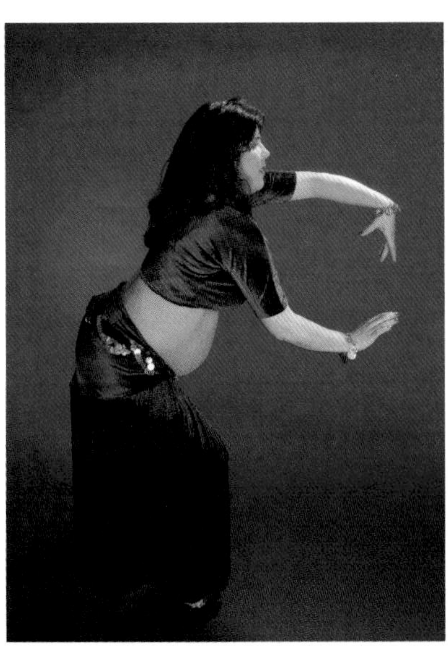

DANCING WITH SNAKE ARMS

When you feel you have mastered snake arms, try bringing them into your dance practice. You can do just about anything with strong snake arms. Try stepping forward on your right foot into a deep lunge, while your arms are snaking to your sides. When you have reached the deepest part of your lunge, hold it and slowly bring your snaking arms forward so that your hands are crossing in front of you. Snake in this position for a few moments, then slowly move your arms back to your sides and slightly behind you. Step back from your lunge, stop snaking and slowly bring your arms to the front in prayer position.

LEGS AND FEET: BASIC STANCES

There are two basic methods of standing in belly dance, and the steps on the following pages should be practiced using both methods. You can either dance with your feet flat on the ground or high on the ball, also called releve.

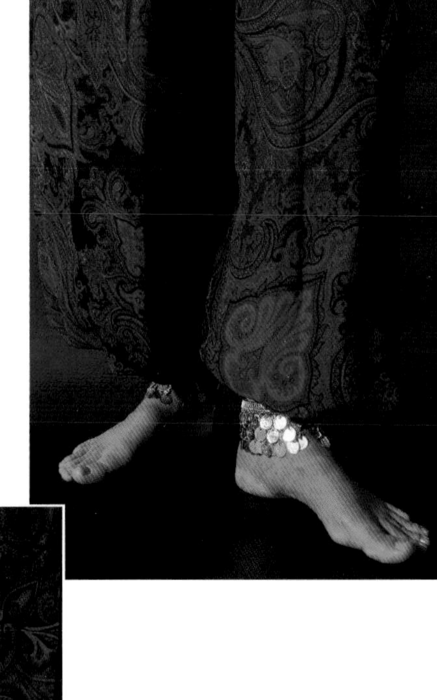

FLAT FOOT

The flat foot position is just what it sounds like. Stand with your entire foot flat on the floor and your body weight equally distributed.

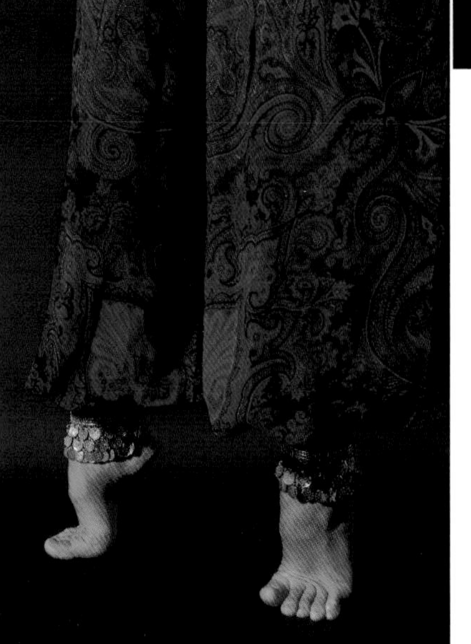

RELEVE

In the releve, or arched foot position, stand high on the ball of the foot with your heels off the ground as if you were stretching up to reach something. All your weight is supported by the ball of the foot and the joints of your first two toes. Very different from the "on points" position in ballet when the dancer stands on the tips of her toes, releve offers more security and stability.

PRACTICE

To practice the releve position, stand with your feet flat and parallel. Raise your heels off the ground until your feet are fully arched and hold for five seconds. Relax and repeat three times more.

Rise up on your heels again and hold the position for two minutes or as long as you can manage. You might find your calves tire after only 30 seconds, so stop when you need to. Your ankles may feel very weak, but this is normal at first so don't worry unless you're in any pain – if you are, stop. The muscles are simply weak and need to be developed. Keep practicing and your calves and ankles will quickly become stronger.

Although many dancers like to wear fashionable high-heeled shoes, I feel these are out of place in most forms of belly dancing. Dancing in releve (right) adds the same height and elegance as high heels and is more in keeping with belly dancing's historic natural roots.

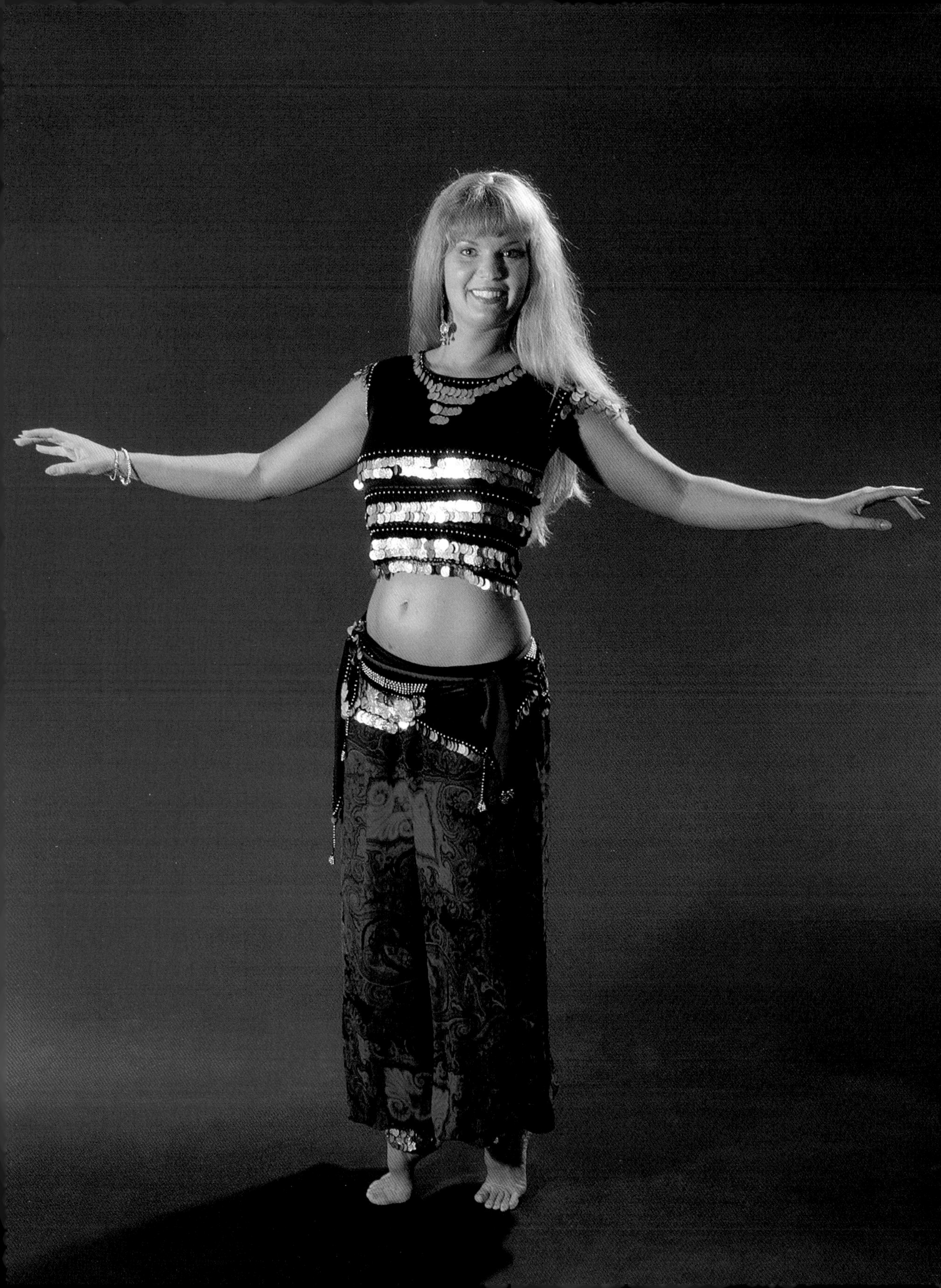

THE BASIC WALK

Simple and classy, the basic walk is the fastest and most graceful way to make an entrance. When walking normally, your heel touches the ground before the rest of your foot. In a belly dance walk it is the opposite – you place your toes on the ground first.

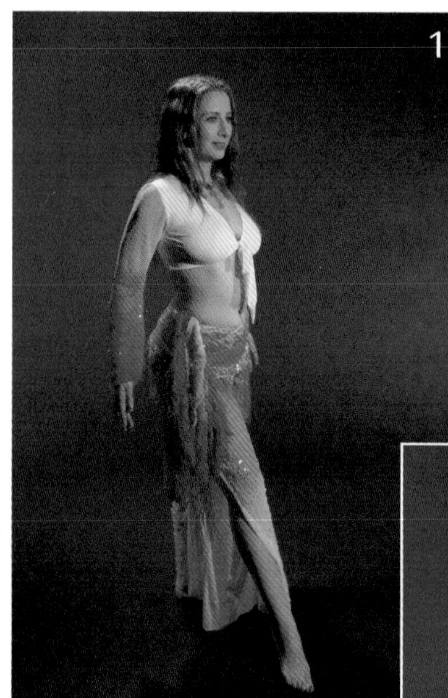
1

1 Stand with your arms at your sides and your feet parallel to one another, 15cm (6in) apart. Lift your right foot 10cm (4in) off the ground and glide it forward.

2 Place your toes on the floor first, followed by your heel.

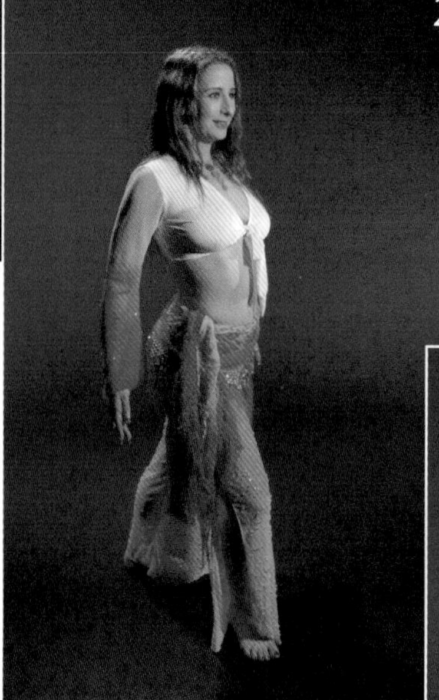
2

3 Repeat with your left foot, touching toes down first as before. Continue, alternating left and right. Lift your chin slightly and walk as smoothly as you can, without too much head bobbing, around your space.

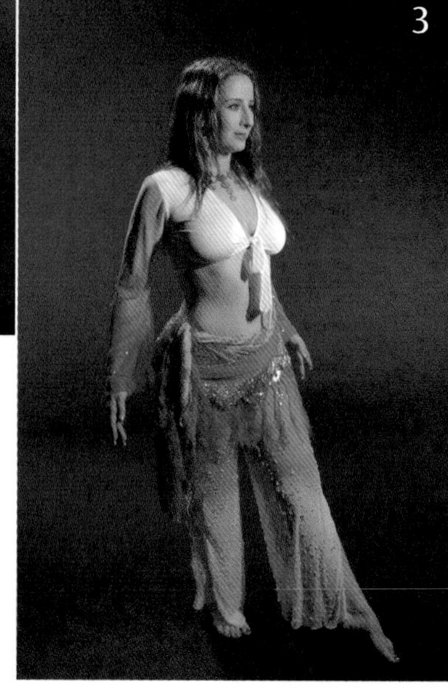
3

ADDING ARMS

There are no particular arm movements associated with this walk. You can simply keep your arms in basic or do something much more complex, such as alternating snake arms (p.55). Experiment and do what works for you.

PHARONIC WALK

If you're in the mood for drama when entering the dance space, try the pharonic walk. An interpretation of postures depicted in Ancient Egyptian hieroglyphics, it conveys a sense of grandeur – of a queen or goddess entering the room.

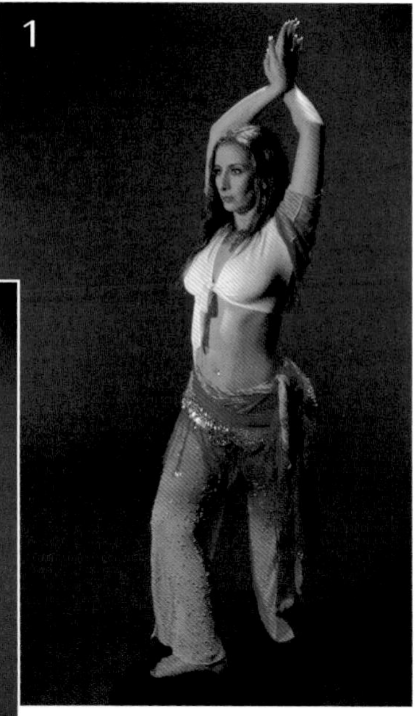

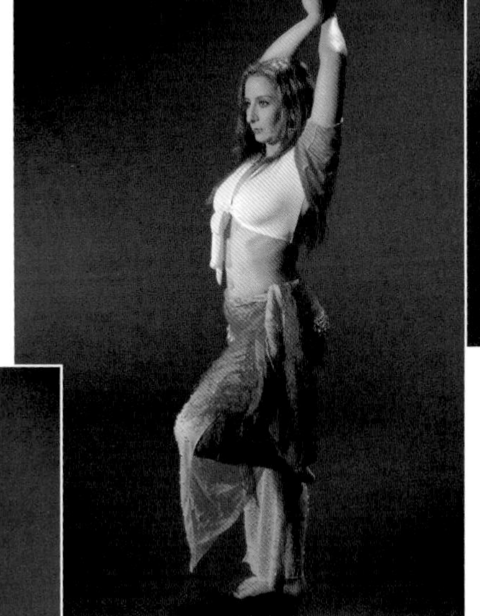

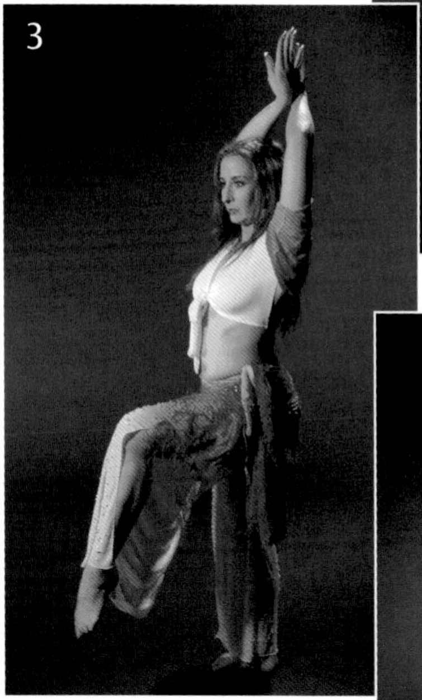

3

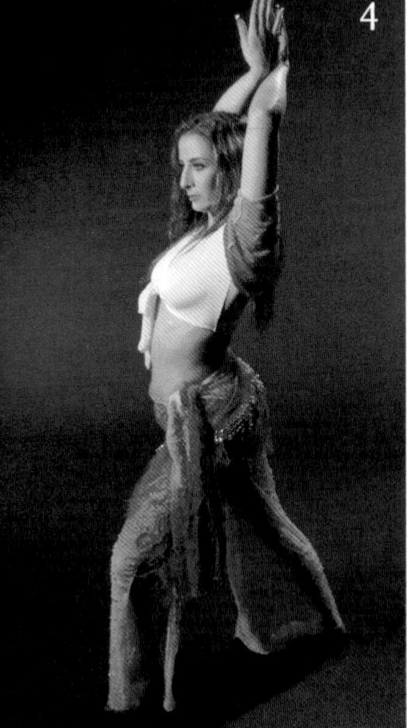

1 Stand with your right side at a 45-degree angle to the front and your head held up. Raise your arms above your head. Cross your hands at the wrists so your palms meet in prayer position.

2 Pointing your toes, lift your left knee until your foot is almost level with your right knee.

3 Slowly and deliberately extend and straighten your leg and place your foot flat on the floor, toes first.

4 Repeat, stepping and lifting your right leg.

PRACTICE

Walk slowly and deliberately, taking time and care with each step, until you reach the center of the dance space.

THE INDIE CROSS STEP

This walk has its origins in ethnic artistic expression – there are many statues of Indian gods and goddesses portrayed as moving in a cross step. Because there are two full steps to each movement, the Indie cross step can be danced with two or four counts. We'll begin with four.

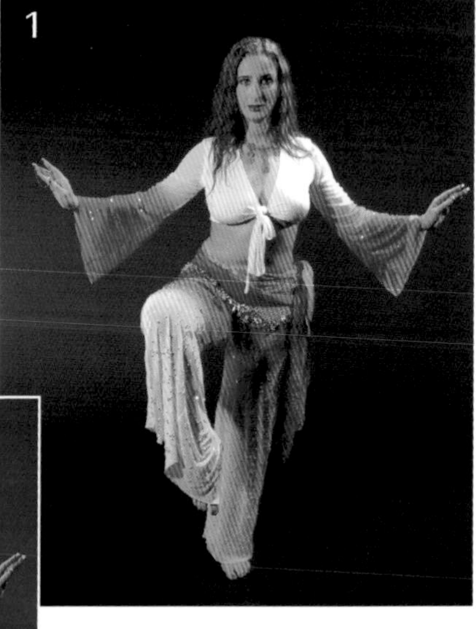

1 Lift your right leg, bending at the knee and toes pointed, to the side so that it is directly under your right arm. Swing your leg over the left and step to the far left across your body for two counts.

2 Transfer your weight onto the right leg by leaning slightly forward for another two counts.

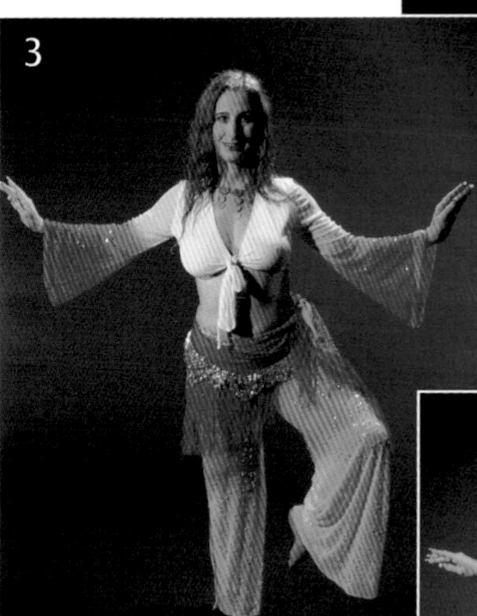

3 Next, lift your left leg to the side and swing it over the right for two counts.

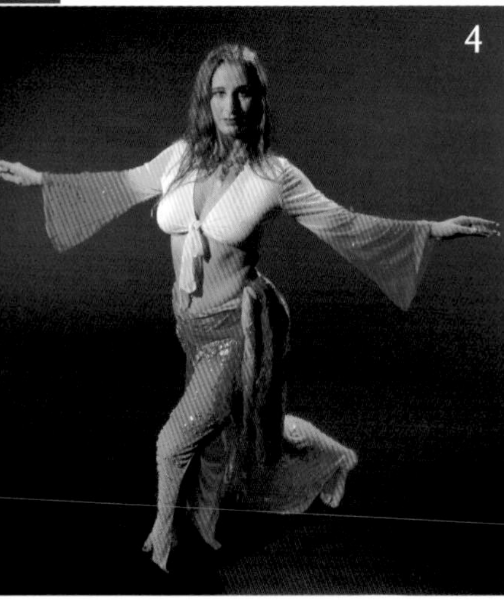

4 Step far right until you can lean and transfer your weight to the left foot for the final two counts.

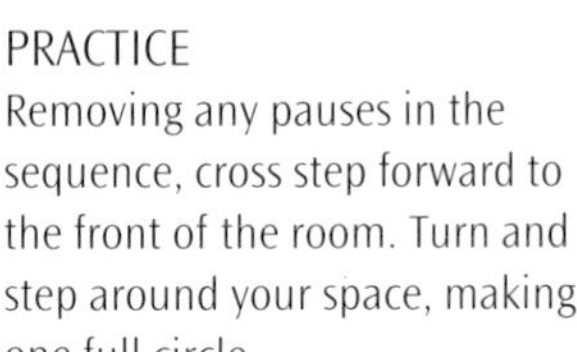

PRACTICE

Removing any pauses in the sequence, cross step forward to the front of the room. Turn and step around your space, making one full circle.

ADDING ARMS

As you step with your right foot, slowly make a left snake arm (p.54) until your weight is completely forward. When stepping to the left, slowly make a right snake arm until your weight is completely forward.

GHAWAZEE SLIDE STEP

Based on three movements and four counts, this is a playful, fast-moving ghawazee (or gypsy) step, which can be used as a travelling step and/or hip step.

1 Lift your right leg and step forward about 60cm (2ft).

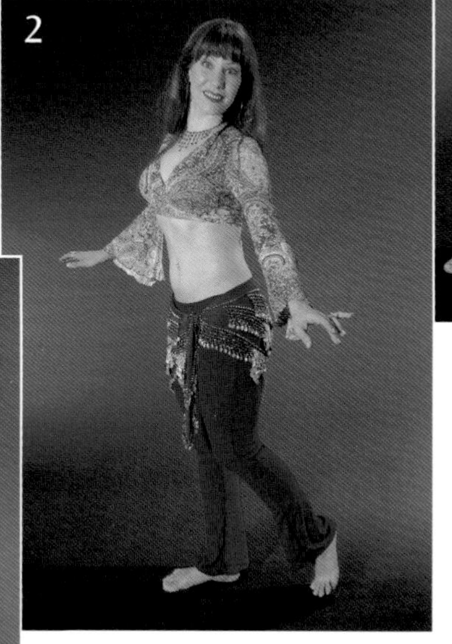

2 Shift your body weight onto your right foot. Steps 1 and 2 should total only one count.

3 Slide your left foot forward until it is about 10cm (4in) behind your right heel for count two.

4 Finally, for count three, transfer your weight onto your back foot, then step forward again with your right foot. Pause for the fourth count.

Beginning another four counts, step forward with your left foot, passing the right. Glide your right foot 7.5–10cm (3–4in) forward to your left, and then step forward again with your left foot. Repeat the entire movement from step 1.

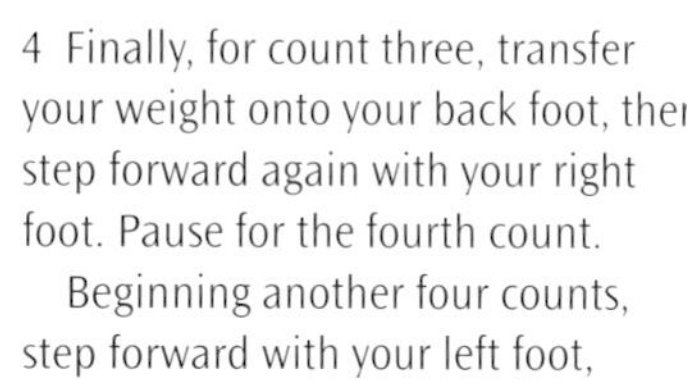

PRACTICE

The way to learn this step is practice. Keep repeating with alternating feet, slowly gaining in speed until you look as if you're skipping. Experiment with large and small steps.

DEBKE

A traditional folk dance step, the eight-step full debke traces its roots back to the desert tribes, who used it as part of their cultural celebrations.

1 Using one count for each step, begin by crossing your left foot in front of your right, stepping almost parallel to your current stance.

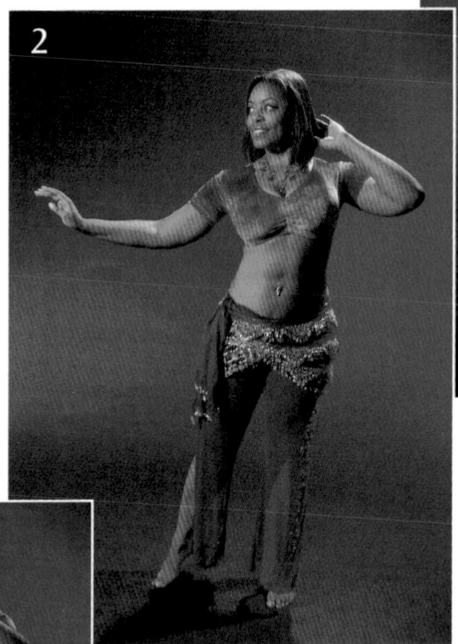

2 Then with your right foot, step directly sideways to the right.

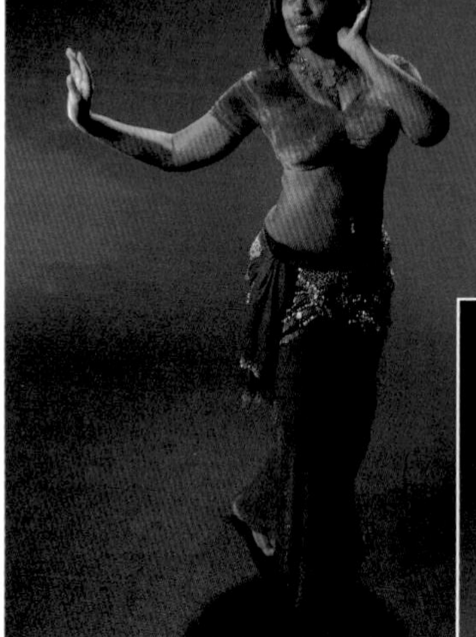

3 With your left foot, now cross behind your right, stepping parallel.

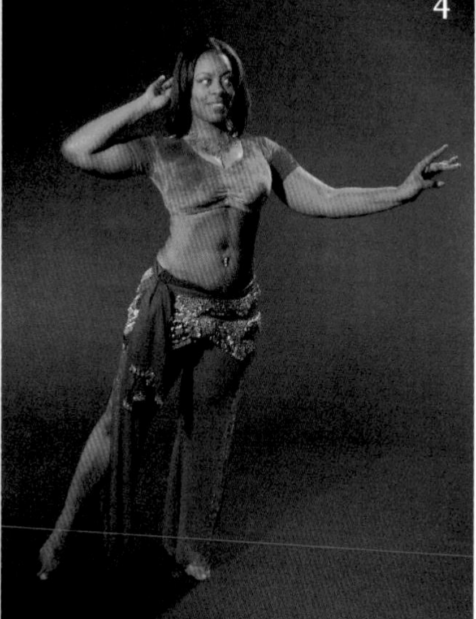

4 Step one more time to the right with your right foot. Touch the floor lightly with the tip of your toe. This sequence should take four counts.

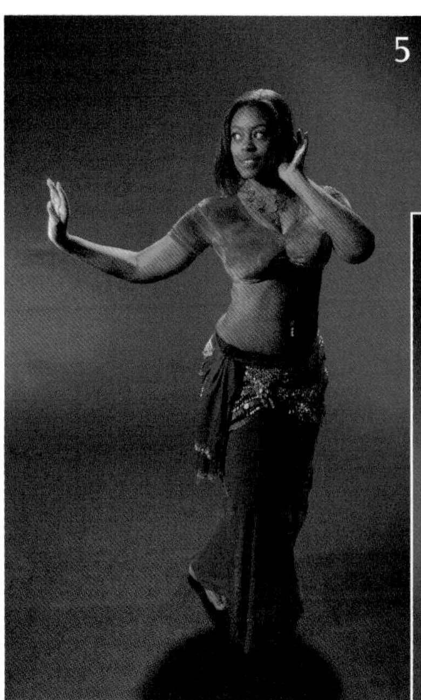

5 Cross your right foot over your left, stepping almost parallel.

6 With your left foot, step directly sideways to the left.

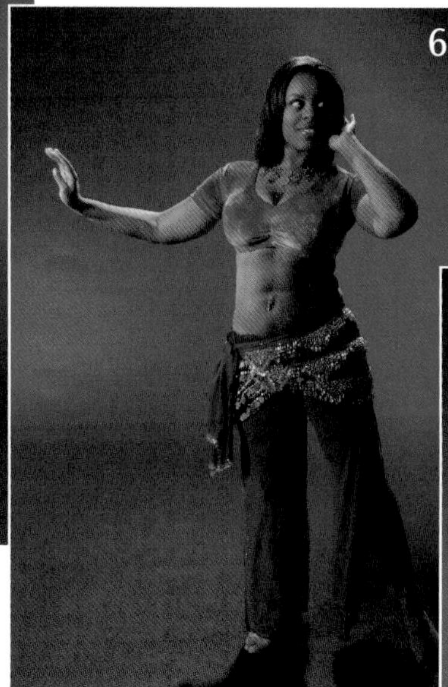

7 With your right foot, step behind your left.

8 With your left foot, step again to the left, touching the floor lightly with the tip of your toe. This sequence should take up the final four counts. Start again at step 1.

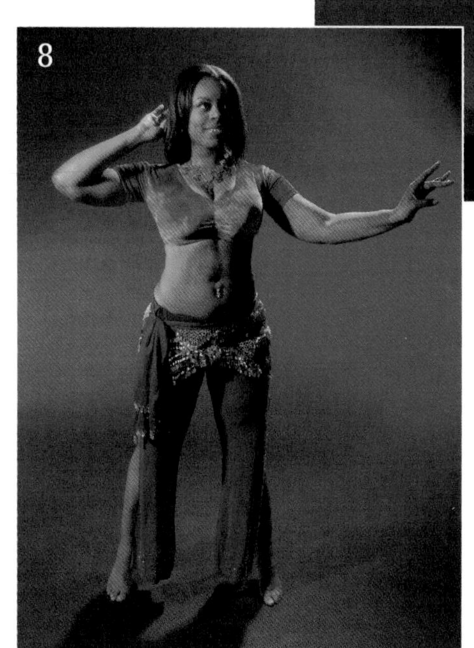

ADDING ARMS

For a fun experiment, raise your arms, bending at the elbows until your hands are parallel to your head. Bend your wrists until your palms are flat and facing the ceiling. When stepping to the left, look in that direction and, keeping your arms stiff, raise your right arm about 7.5cm (3in) higher than your left.

When you step to the right, return your right arm to its original level and raise the left while looking right.

PRACTICE

Perform the full debke right and left and then try it forward in each direction on the diagonal right and left. Try holding your arms in a variety of positions – be as creative as you want.

KASHLIMAR

Also a traditional folk step, the kashlimar can be performed in one place or used to travel across your dance space. Each step in the sequence is equal to one count.

1 Step forward with your right foot. As you transfer your weight forward, lift your left foot slightly off the floor.

2 Now reverse direction and step down with your left foot. Rock back your weight and lift your right foot slightly off the ground. Continue shifting your center of gravity back and step about 60cm (2ft) behind your left foot with your right.

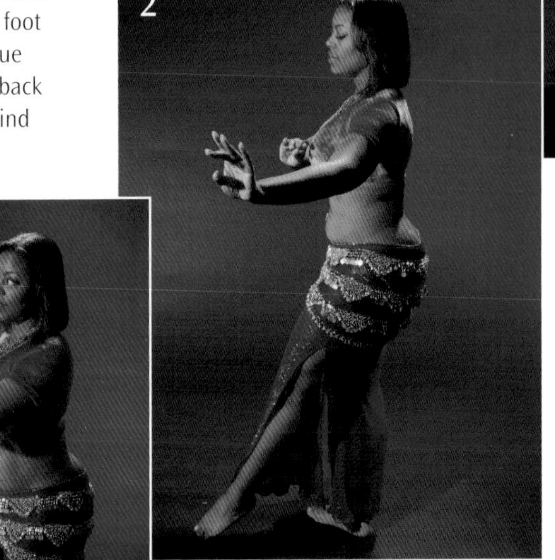

3 When all your weight is on your right leg, lift your left foot slightly. Place it down and rock forward. Transfer your weight to your left leg.

4 Step forward with your right foot until it is back in its original position (see step 1).

PRACTICE

Gently keep the kashlimar step going for eight full repetitions. Then try changing direction by stepping 45 degrees to the right side for four full steps. Step forward and back again for another four, then 45 degrees to the left for four counts.

ADDING ARMS

Easy, relaxed arm movements are best for this gentle travel step. When stepping forward, gently swing your arms to the front, leading with your wrists. When stepping back, gently swing your arms behind you, again leading with your wrists.

FRONT CROSS STEP TURN

1 Again working with four counts, dip down and forward slightly, while stepping 15–30cm (6–12in) across your right foot with your left. Rise high onto the ball of your right foot. Begin an ascending snake arm (p.54) on the right, leading with your elbow toward the ceiling and keeping your left arm in basic.

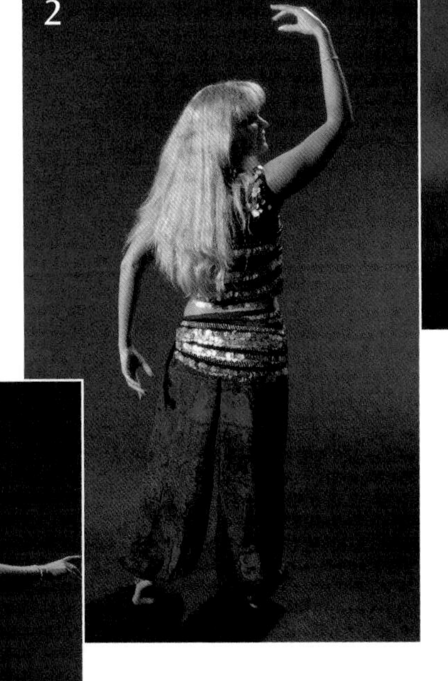

2 Pivot on both feet until you are facing the back of the room with your right arm high above your head, still leading with your elbow.

3 Lower your right arm and lift your left, continuing to lead with your elbows back to basic. With your left foot, quickly step across your right, pivoting until you are once more facing the front of your dance space.

4 Begin a descending right snake arm and an ascending left, at the same time pivoting on your feet until you are once more facing front. Most of your weight should be on your left leg. Follow through and finish your arm movements on the left and right.

PRACTICE

Repeat back and forth four times on each side or until you feel secure. If you begin losing your balance, don't worry – you're just getting dizzy. Take a break and try again later.

THREE-POINT TURN

This turn is danced with two or four counts, even though it is three steps. Unlike the cross step turn (p.65), which is on the spot, this turn moves you a few feet in each direction. Start slowly. Try four-counts, then speed up to two.

1 Begin count one by stepping out 60–90cm (2–3ft) to the right with your right leg.

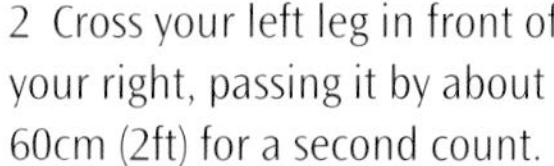

2 Cross your left leg in front of your right, passing it by about 60cm (2ft) for a second count.

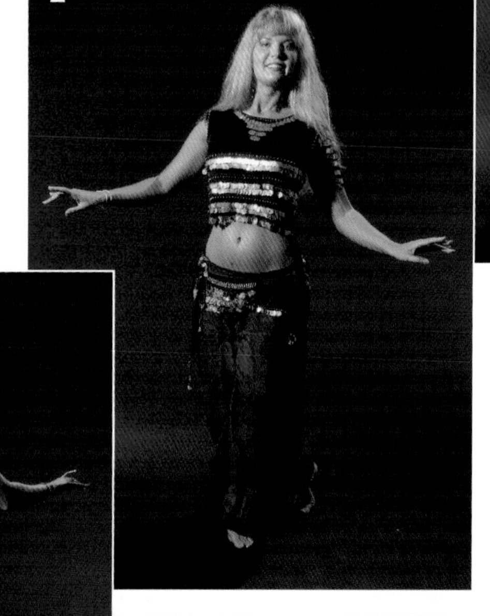

3 As you place your left foot down, pivot on your feet until you are facing the back of your dance space.

4 Sweep your right leg behind your left, passing it by about 60cm (2ft). As you place your right leg down, simultaneously pivot on your feet until you are facing the front of the room again for count three. Pause for the fourth count, then try a three-point to the left.

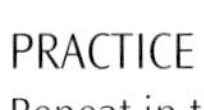

PRACTICE

Repeat in the opposite direction, now stepping left, right, left. Try the turns with some spotting (p.27) so you don't get too dizzy.

ADDING ARMS

Add arm movements by bringing your arms together at chest level as you pivot to the back of the room, and separating them when you return to face front.

THREE-POINT DROP

I love this step. It reminds me of dramatic dance scenes in Hollywood movies of the 1940s, when temple priestesses are shown dancing seductively for their goddess, unaware that they are being spied upon by scoundrels or thieves.

1 Start by following the steps for a basic three-point turn to the right. On the last step, as you place your right foot down, transfer 70 percent of your body weight onto it.

2 Bend your knee and slide your left foot away from you so that you are in a full lunge supported by your right leg. Drop your head gently but fully forward. Sweep your left arm down in front until your palm is on the floor. Simultaneously swing your right arm high up behind you. This slide and drop replaces the fourth beat pause in the original turn.

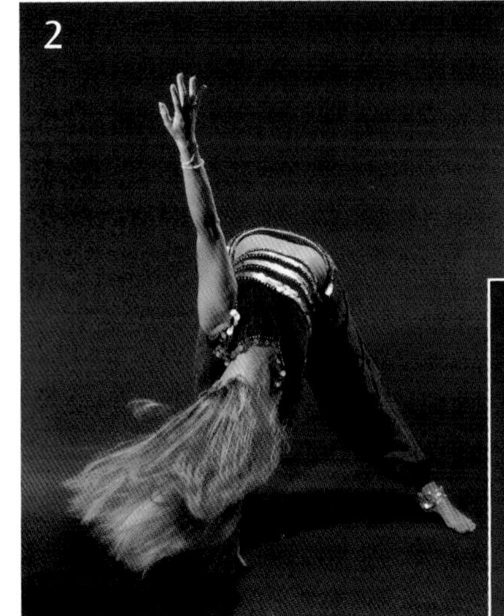

3 Then taking a full four counts, flip your head up and peer straight ahead, while slowly beginning to rise from the lunge.

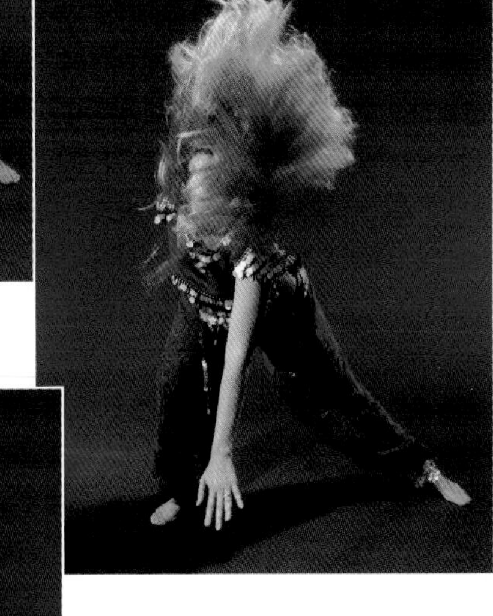

4 To come up, gradually lower your right arm. At the same time, drag your left foot in to meet your right while straightening your right knee, until you are back to your starting position. Repeat this in the other direction, lunging onto the left foot and sliding back with the right. Your right arm should be forward, with your hand touching the ground, while your left is raised straight up behind your body. Rise up slowly as before, gradually dropping your left arm and sliding your right foot in.

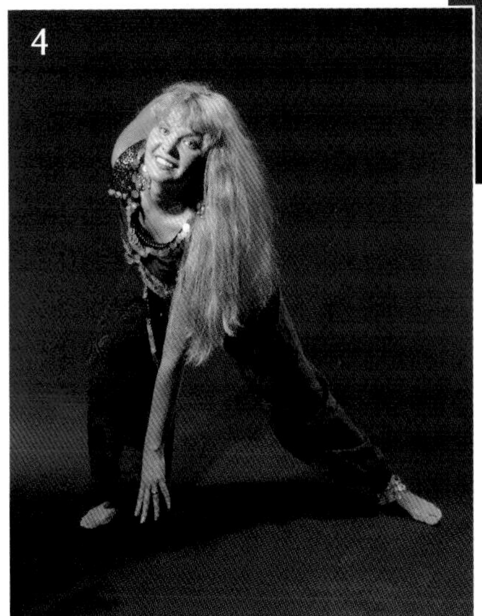

PRACTICE

Repeat six times, alternating turn by turn, left and right.

ACCENTUATING THE FACE

The quick flip of the head in this step is a perfect chance to convey different feelings and expressions. Experiment, just for fun. As you lift your head dramatically from the drop, try looking very serious for one lift, then joyful for the next. Maybe you can put a gleam of mischief in your eye or even a look of shock or dismay.

DERVISH TURN

The whirling dervishes are ceremonial Sufis who split off from traditional Islam sometime in the 13th century. Part of their practice is spinning gracefully in circles, with one palm facing the sky and the other facing the earth. Many people associate the whirling dervish with frantic speed, but the real dervishes start slowly, then build up pace as they whirl. The same is true for this turn. Be prepared to get a little dizzy because you cannot spot (p.27) with this turn!

WARNING
People suffering from neck pain or any spinal condition should not perform the head accents included in this step.

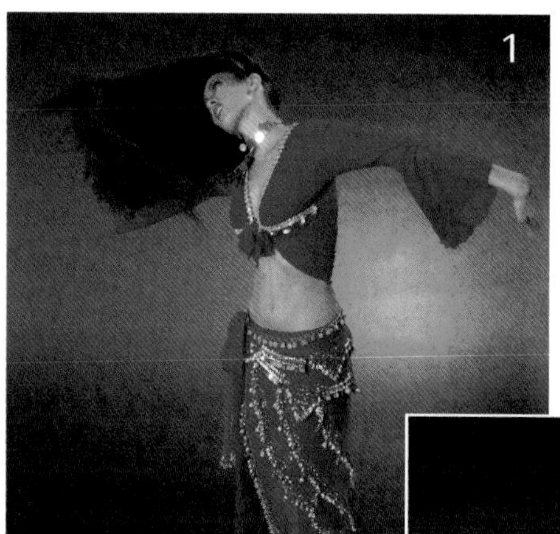

1 Stand with your feet parallel and flat on the ground. Tilt your head slightly to one side and raise your arms to your sides so they are parallel with your shoulders. To start, both hands should be in basic (p.21). Begin spinning slowly and evenly, using small steps. After two rotations, switch your right hand from basic to offering (p.21) and speed up a little.

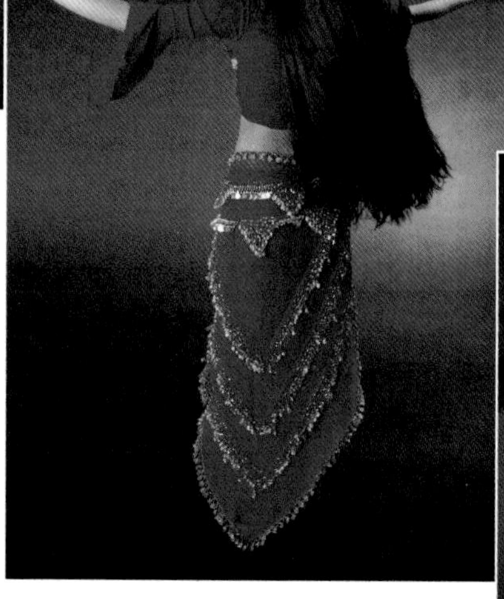

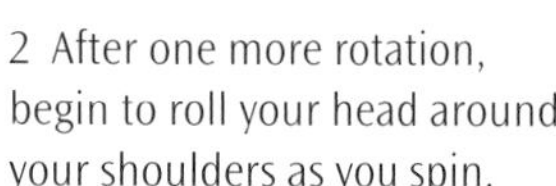

2 After one more rotation, begin to roll your head around your shoulders as you spin.

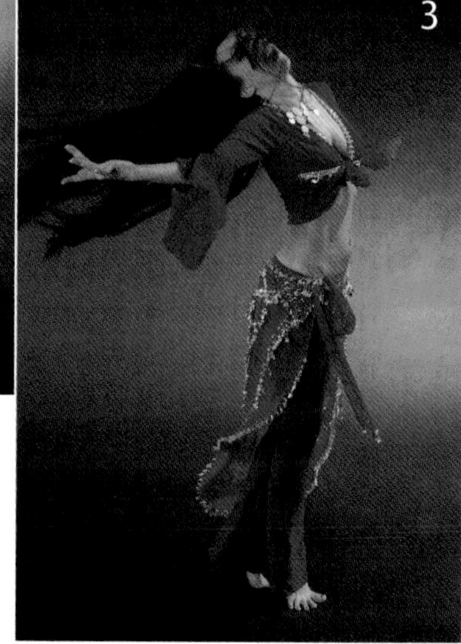

3 If you have long hair and your neck muscles are strong and flexible enough, flip your hair around as your head is circling on your shoulders.

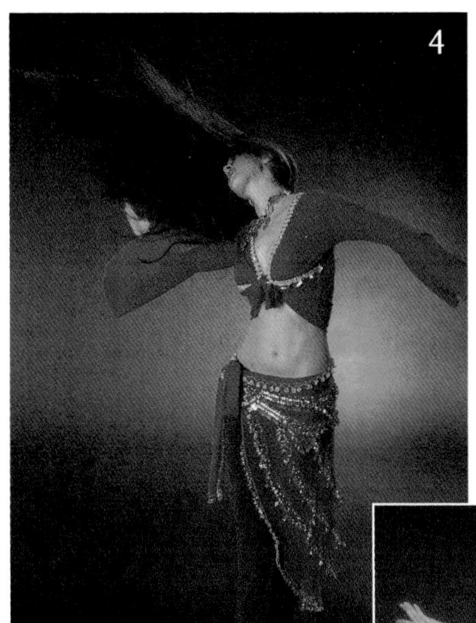

4 Pick up speed until you are whirling very quickly for three or four more rotations. Continue to whip your head and hair around.

5

5 When you are ready to finish the turn, stop rolling your head and slowly come to a halt. As you do so, return your right hand to basic and lower your arms to chest level.

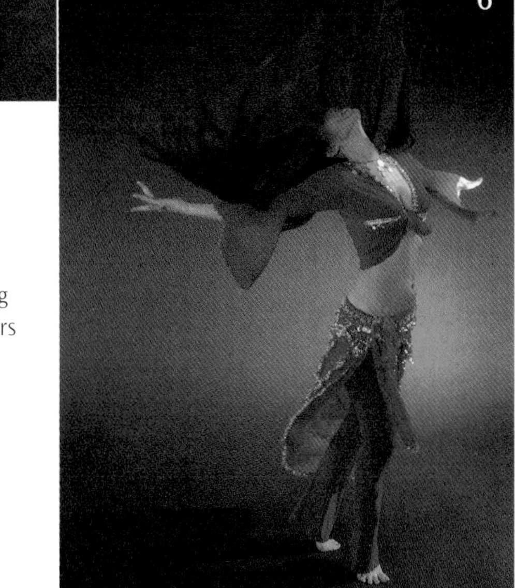

6 Carefully flip your head, tossing your hair back over your shoulders for a terrific finale.

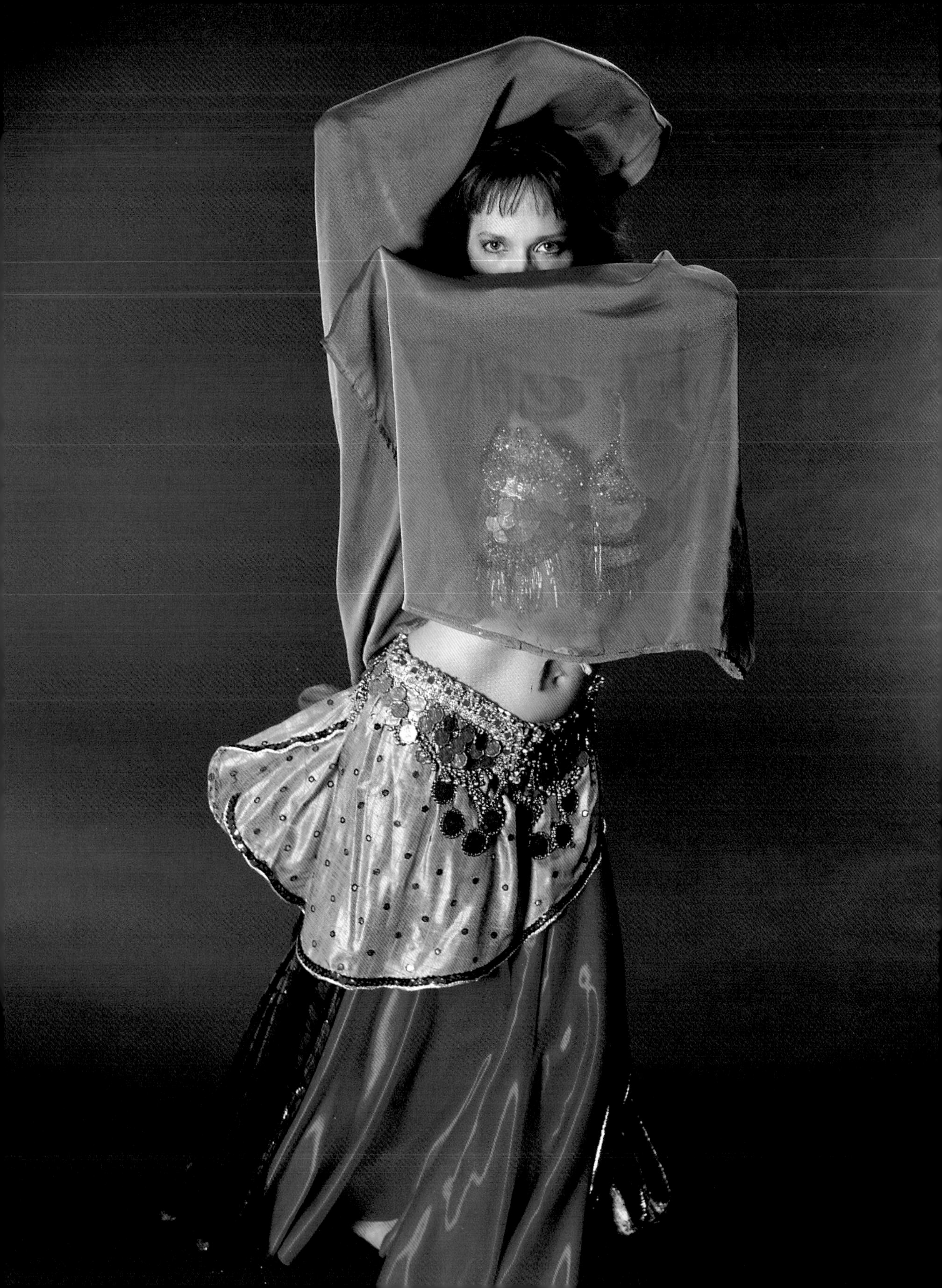

4 Adding mystery

Belly dancers portrayed in films or paintings usually have a veil. Sometimes covering the face or body, sometimes held in the hands, the diaphanous veil seems to defy gravity as it floats about the dancer – a wonderful image that never fails to captivate the observer.

STYLES AND TYPES OF VEIL

Most veils are rectangular, but half-circles and triangles are not uncommon. Veils are generally made from magic silk, silk chiffon or polyester chiffon, but almost any fabric can be used provided it is light and beautiful. Veils can be very simple or decorated with complex sequin and bead designs.

CHOOSING THE VEIL THAT'S RIGHT FOR YOU

Try to choose a veil that looks good with whatever you like to dance in but is not exactly the same colour. It should be significantly lighter or darker so that it contrasts with your clothes or costume and doesn't get lost. Deep shades like burgundy or royal purple are wonderful if you're feeling moody and serious, while delicate pastels and springtime shades are perfect for joyful and spirited dancing.

Next, decide what length of veil will work best for you. Too short a veil restricts the movements you can do with it and interrupts its gentle floating. Too long a veil will drag on the ground, and if you step on it, the smooth fabric will make your feet slide out from under you so fast that you won't know what happened until you're flat on the floor! One handy guide I use for my students and myself is to measure the length of your arms, fingertip to fingertip. Then add on another 90cm (3ft) so that the veil will drape from each fingertip by 45cm (18in). Don't worry if you can't find a veil with the exact measurements; a difference of 5–7.5cm (2–3in) is fine.

The next question is, how much float should the veil have? Which veil you choose depends on how you'd like to use it. Is it purely ornamental or is it an extension of your feelings and body? In Egyptian belly dancing, which is primarily cabaret style, the dancers generally enter with a veil, spend a few minutes or so dancing with it, then discard it to continue their routine. When a dancer plans on using a veil like this, a highly ornate veil is a good choice and it can be made of heavier, highly decorated fabric. Since the dancer isn't really using the veil much, the increased weight won't disturb her routine.

However, I'd like to encourage you to use the veil more fully, so you may want to choose something light and airy for your first veil. If you're purchasing a veil, throw the fabric high into the air and without letting it go, allow it to float down. The veil that takes the longest to sink is the right one!

THE BEAUTY OF THE VEIL

I consider the veil to be an integral part of the dance, adding incredible beauty and feeling. Don't be surprised if you fall in love with veil work and become afflicted with "veilitis". This is a condition that only affects belly dancers, compelling them to buy veils in all their favourite colours until their wardrobes are exploding in rainbows. There is no known cure except lack of storage space!

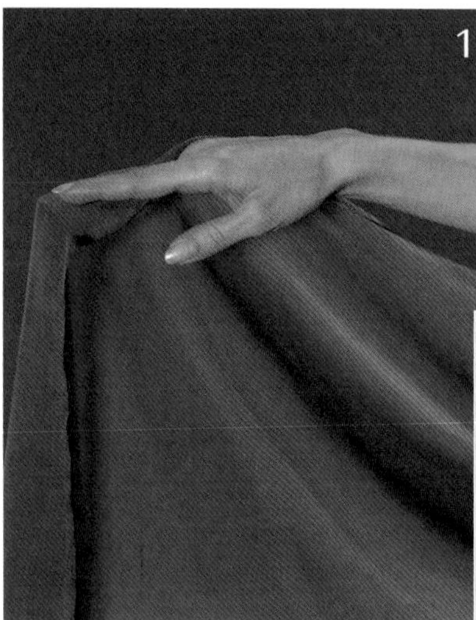

HOW TO HOLD A VEIL

1 Grasp the veil draped behind you, with an even amount of fabric cascading from your hands on each side. Hold your right hand in basic one position (p.21) and drape the veil over your last three fingers, while threading it between your index and middle finger.

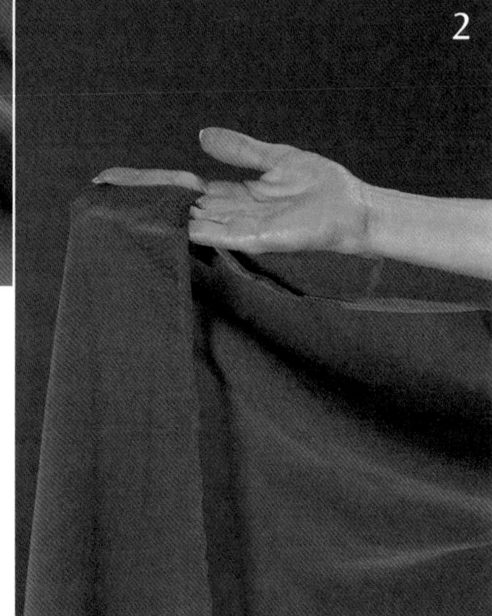

2 Experiment with different hand positions to help get a feel for dancing with the veil.

MAKING A VEIL

Making your own veil is easy and gives a wonderful personal touch to your costume. Take your measurements (p.71), pop into your local fabric supplier and ask to see some silk or polyester chiffon. Select the colour you like, unroll a length or two and wave it about to see how light it is and how well it floats. Don't be shy! The fabric that is the lightest is the best choice. Ask for the fabric to be cut, rather than torn, which can cause pulls in the body of the fabric and fray the edges.

To seam your veil, fold each edge over by 5mm (¼in) and press with a warm iron. Fold over another 5mm (¼in) and press again so that you have fully rolled hems. With a needle and thread or sewing machine, stitch along the middle of the hems to secure them. Press the entire veil once more and you are ready to start dancing.

BODY GLIMPSING

Body glimpsing is a way of using the veil to reveal parts of the body briefly, then hide them again, giving the impression of letting someone in on a secret. This technique can be used to focus on any one part of your body at a time.

1 Cascade the veil round you by quickly crossing your arms in front of your chest, enclosing your body.

2 Quickly unfurl the veil and leading with your elbows and wrists, raise both arms above your head. Perform a quick high and low undulation.

3 Rapidly close the veil across your chest again and turn your body to the right.

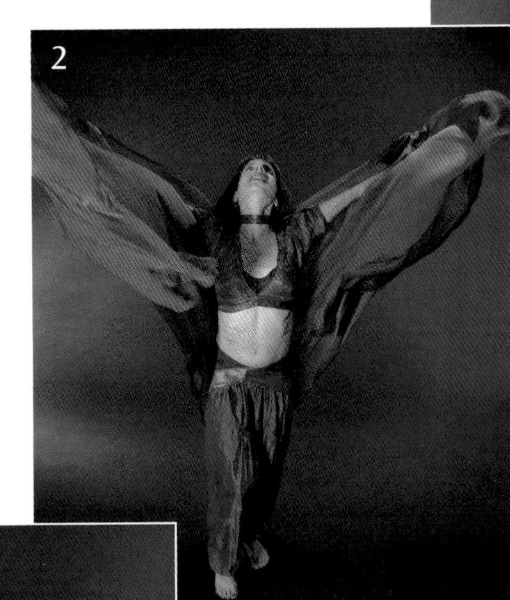

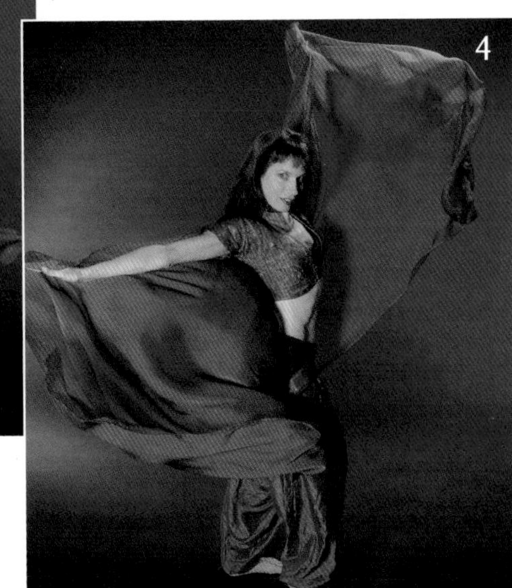

4 Open the veil, leading with your elbows and wrists, but this time lower your right arm and raise your left. Dance six hip drops on the right side. Close the veil and turn to face the left. Open your veil as in step 2, but with your left arm up and right arm low. Dance one hip thrust, forward and back, then wrap yourself in the veil again.

WAYS OF WEARING YOUR VEIL

In a full routine, the veil dance is not usually performed until the second or third piece of music. Instead of having to interrupt her dance to fetch the veil, a belly dancer carries her veil draped around her body until she needs it – a practice called "wrapping". Wraps should be simple and allow for unrestricted movement as well as easy unwrapping. As you learn to wrap your veil, let it drape in loose folds like a flowing waterfall of fabric. Make sure no part of the veil is hanging on the floor where it could cause you to slip and fall.

THE BASIC WRAP

1 With the veil behind you, take the left side and tuck a part of it into your right shoulder strap or sleeve.

2 Take the right side and tuck part of that into your left shoulder strap or sleeve. The veil will be wrapped loosely round your waist and crossed over your chest, with the excess fabric hanging from your shoulders.

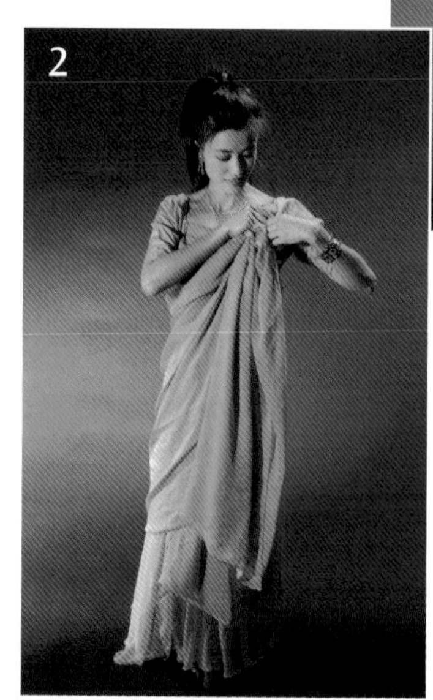

THE TOGA

1 Hold the veil in front of you. With your right hand, tuck the veil inside your costume at your right hip. Make sure nothing is dragging on the floor on that side.

2 With your left hand, wrap the veil behind you and pass it to your right hand. Bring the veil under your right arm and tuck the remaining length of fabric into your left shoulder strap.

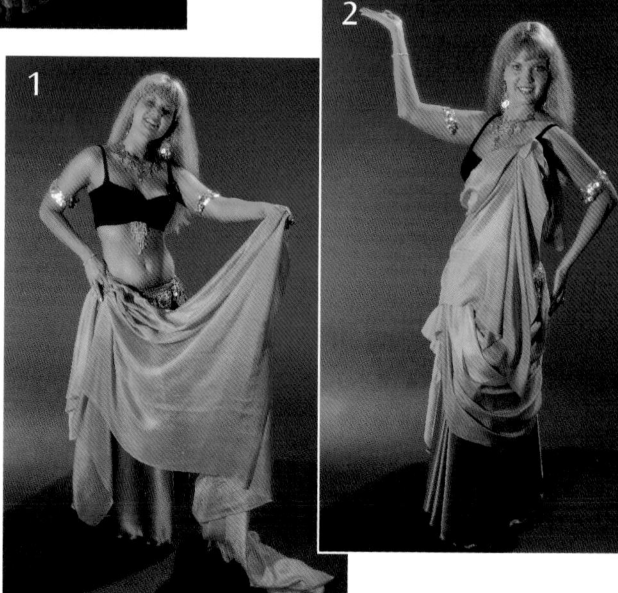

THE GODDESS

1 Hold the veil in front of you and with your right hand, tuck it inside your costume at your right hip.

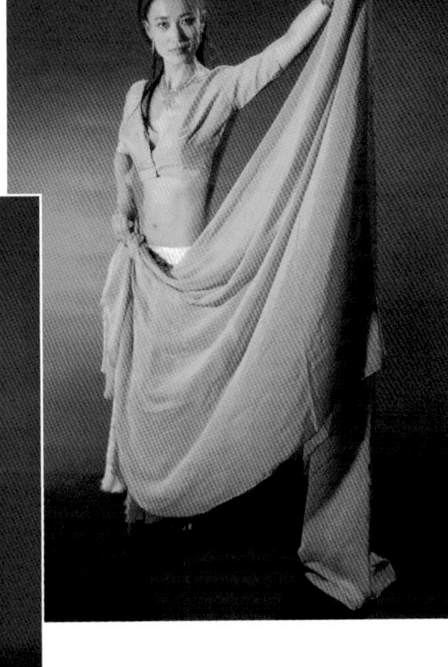

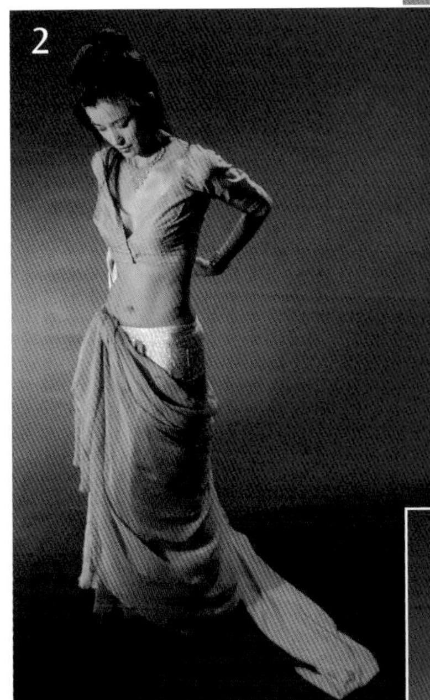

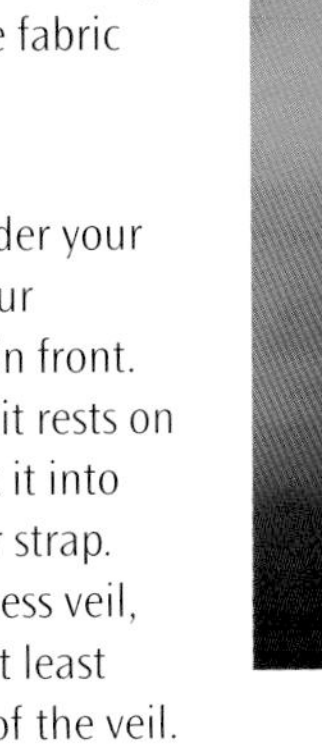

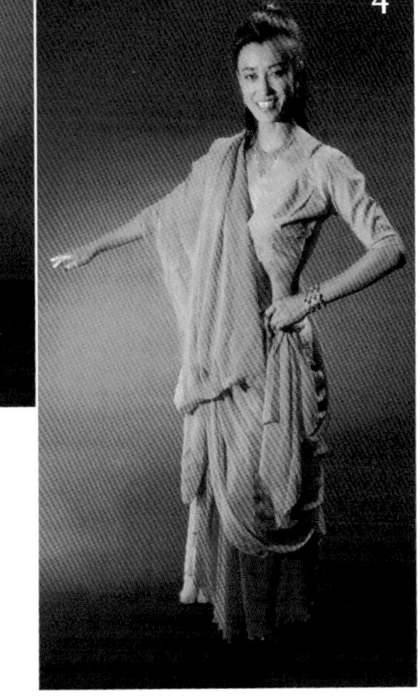

2 As you did with the toga, take the veil in your left hand and wrap it behind you, passing the fabric into your right hand.

3 Instead of bringing the veil under your right arm, bring it up and over your shoulder. Allow it to drape down in front. Take a small bit of the veil where it rests on the top of your shoulder and tuck it into the top of your sleeve or shoulder strap. With your left hand, grasp the excess veil, which is hanging down in front, at least 30cm (12in) up from the bottom of the veil.

4 Tuck the veil that you are holding in your left hand into the front of your costume on the left side, by your belly. With your right hand, do the same with the excess veil on your right side. The veil will billow out from your waist and hang in gentle waves.

THE SEDUCTION OF UNVEILING

Unveiling is one of the most sensuous elements of belly dancing. But it needs to be performed with great care and elegance if it is to convey sensuality rather than overt sexuality. Classic dancers and appreciative viewers prefer the gentle delicacy of a caress across the cheek rather than an jarring slap across the face, so to speak.

UNVEILING IN A SPIN

A pleasingly subtle method of unveiling is to unwrap while spinning. This technique takes time and skill to master but is well worth it. There are only two rules to follow when learning this technique: first, never look at your veil or your hands; second, only one hand at a time should be used to untuck your veil. The technique is shown here with the toga wrap, but any of the styles shown on pp.74–75 can be unwrapped in a spin.

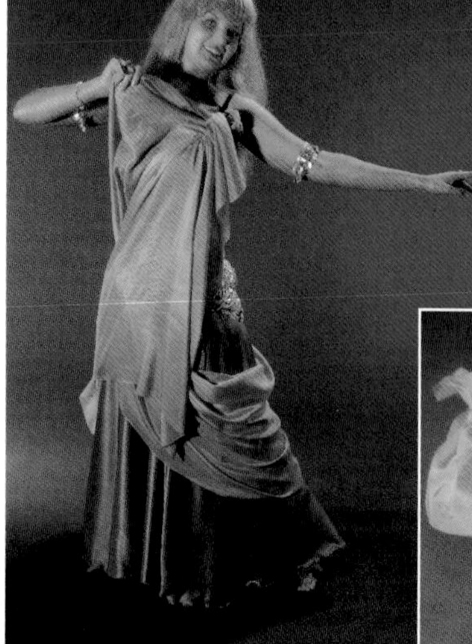

1 Begin by reminding yourself of the last point where your veil is tucked in. Start slowly spinning with small steps, as if you were dancing a dervish turn.

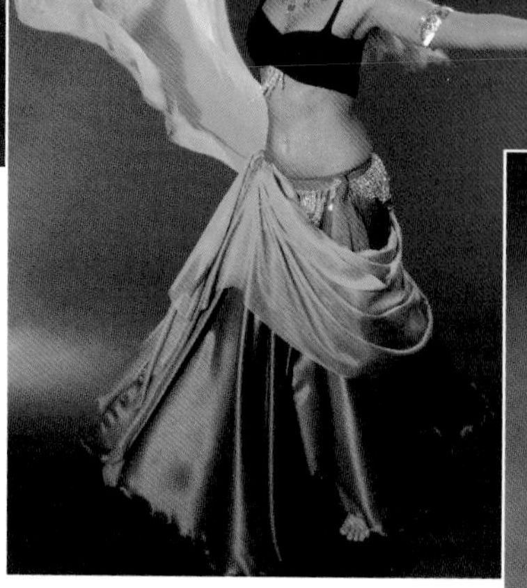

2 Languidly grab the veil at the last tuck point and gently, without looking, pull the veil straight out from the tuck.

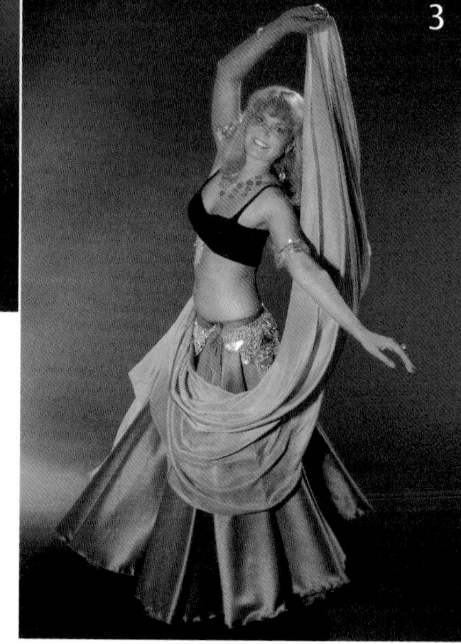

3 Little by little, continue unwrapping by pulling the veil from each point while spinning.

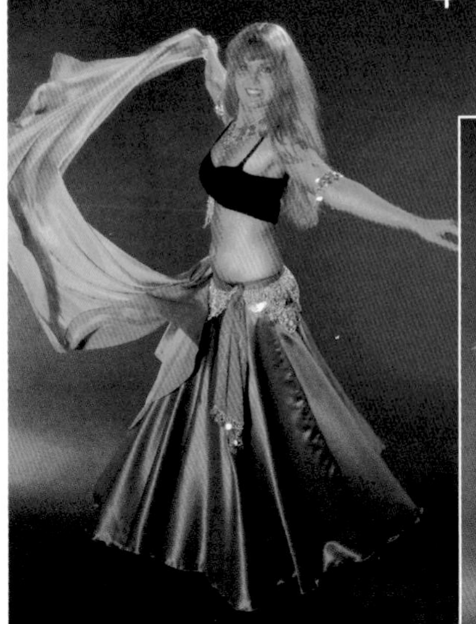

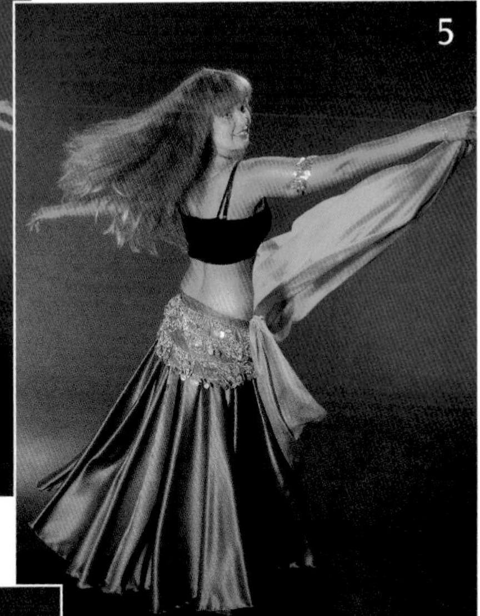

4, 5 Depending on how you tucked the veil, you may need to switch it to the other hand, toss it over your shoulder or even swirl it round your head.

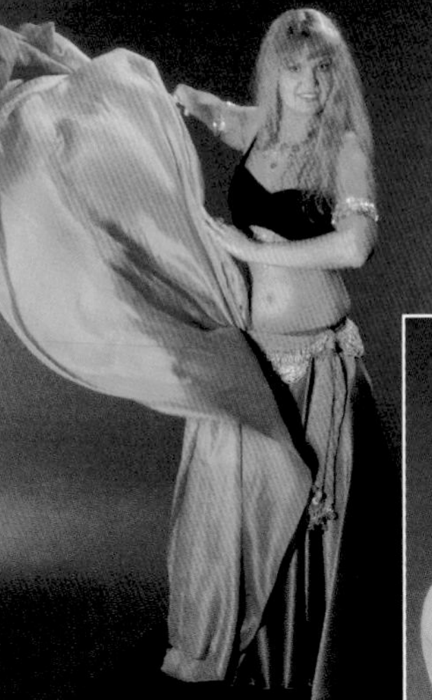

6 When the veil is at its last tuck point, keep spinning and grab it with your free hand. Gently pull it free.

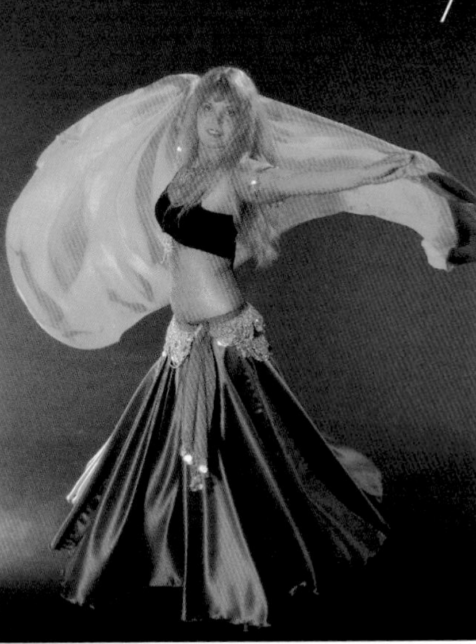

7 Remain spinning and manipulating the veil until there is the same amount of veil on each side. Slowly come to a halt and pose until you gather your dizzy wits from all that turning!

UNVEILING IN STEPS

If you find the unveiling spin (pp.76–77) a bit overwhelming, try unveiling in steps. The technique is not just to pull out the tucks one at a time while standing in place, but to unveil step by step in between some elegant dance movements.

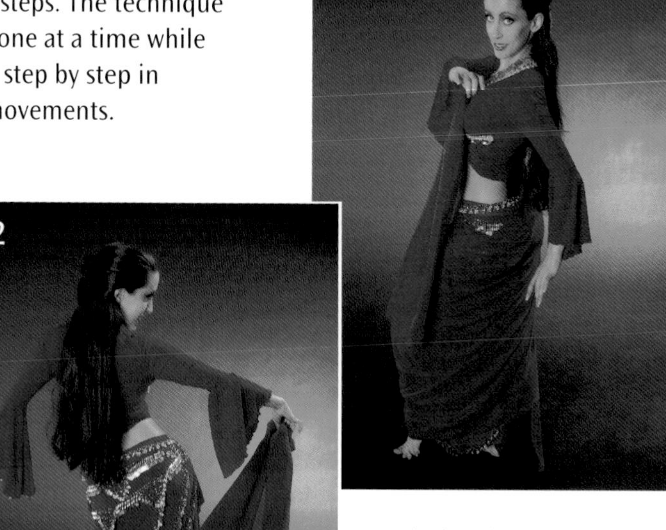

PART ONE: CREATING A SAIL

1 The technique is shown here using the toga wrap but is possible with any of the veil wrap styles on pages 74–75. With your back facing the front of your dance space, begin hip rolling (p.32) left and right. With your right hand, grasp the first tuck point at your shoulder.

2 Slowly pull the veil free from the first tuck point.

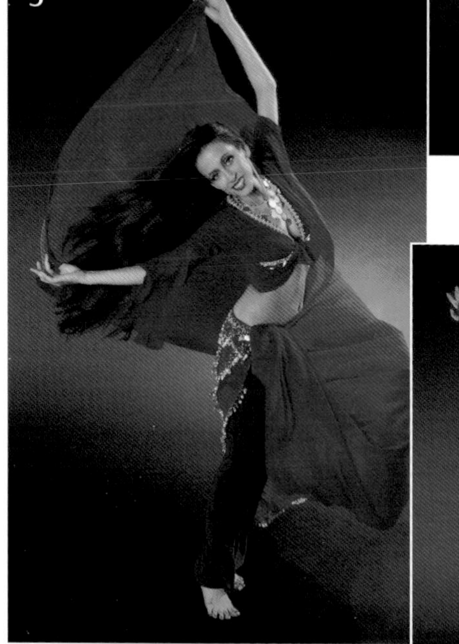

3 Begin unwrapping your body by bringing the veil across your chest to the right. When the veil is directly in front of you, take hold of it in your left hand and adjust it until you have one side in each hand. Raise the veil above your head and lean diagonally to the right while spinning to the left. The veil will catch the air and billow out behind you like a tall sail.

4 Dance two rotations, then switch directions by leaning to the left and spinning to the right. After another two rotations, come to a gentle halt facing front and hold the veil up at an even level behind you.

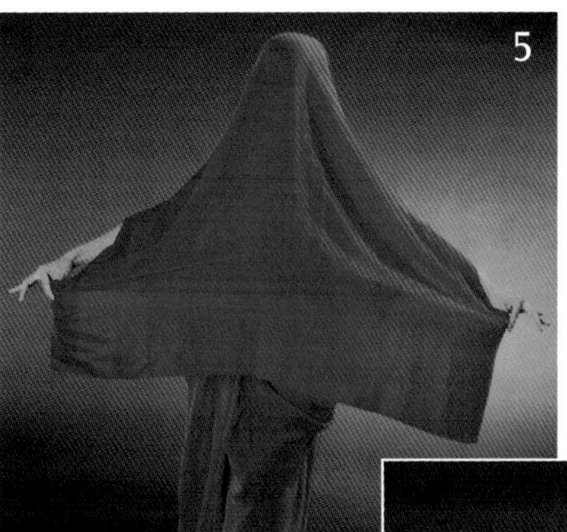

PART TWO: CREATING A TENT

5 With both arms, drape the veil over your head, pulling it gently so that it reaches down to your waist. Since your waist and face can't be seen, this is the chance to peek at where the last tuck point is – but don't move your head.

6 Perform some elegant snake arms (p.54) or perhaps a shimmy (p.38) and a few reverse hip rolls (p.33) until you're sure of the position of the last tuck point.

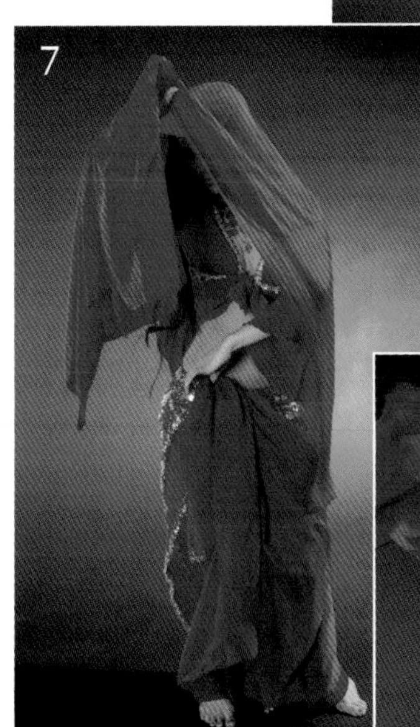

7 Turn your back to the front of the room again and with your left hand grab the veil at your waist. Reach your right arm over your face to take hold of the veil from its left side. (Although the dancer here is shown facing the front to demonstrate what is happening, this step should always be performed with your back to the audience so no one can see how you magically unveil.)

8 Holding the veil securely, spin one rotation and pull the veil free. You are now dramatically and amazingly unveiled!

UNDERSTANDING LIFT AND CASCADE

These simple veil movements will help you learn how to control your veil so that it flows like a gentle breeze and appears soft as a cloud. Once you understand the nature of lift and cascade, anything is possible.

Unless otherwise indicated, always begin veil steps in basic foundation (p.20), holding the veil behind you.

PREPARATION

Holding the veil firmly in each hand, quickly but gently raise your arms, lifting the veil. Drop them slowly, allowing the veil to gather air and cascade down as it falls. Experiment with the speed of lifting and dropping, while observing how the veil falls and where it catches the most air in relation to how fast you move your arms. The technique is to drop your arms fast enough not to interrupt the fall of the veil, while making sure that they are moving slowly enough not to drag down the material.

LIFT AND CASCADE

1 Leading with your wrists, quickly raise your arms and lift the veil. Just as you reach up as far as you can, flick your wrists to extend your hands upward with a snap. This will kick the veil up another foot or so, giving it more height.

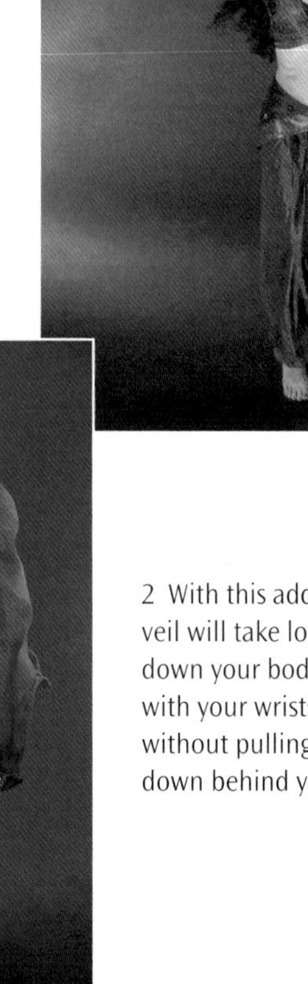

2 With this added height, the veil will take longer to cascade down your body. Again leading with your wrists, gently and without pulling, guide the veil down behind you.

CASCADING BACK AND FORTH

1 Stand with your palms facing up. As you did with the lift and cascade, sweep your arms up above your head. But instead of letting them drop behind you, arc your arms forward, so that they pass over your head to the front of your body, with the veil trailing behind.

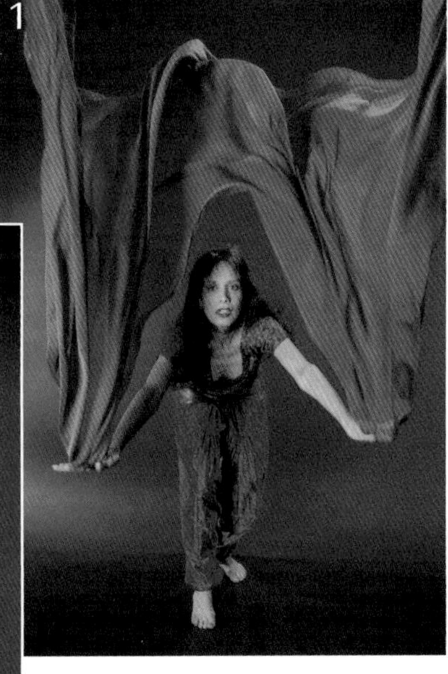

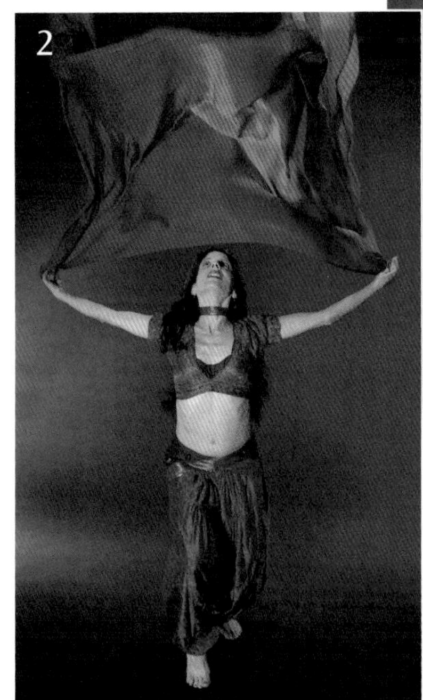

2 Allow your arms to drop at a pace that permits the veil to cascade gently down to the ground. Reverse the sweep without drag or interruption by passing your arms back over your head so that the veil can cascade down behind you again.

PRACTICE

Begin by lifting the veil four times behind you. Follow with another four lifts, including wrist flicks to see how high you can get the veil to go. Then repeat front and back cascades six times and finish with four consecutive left and right cascades.

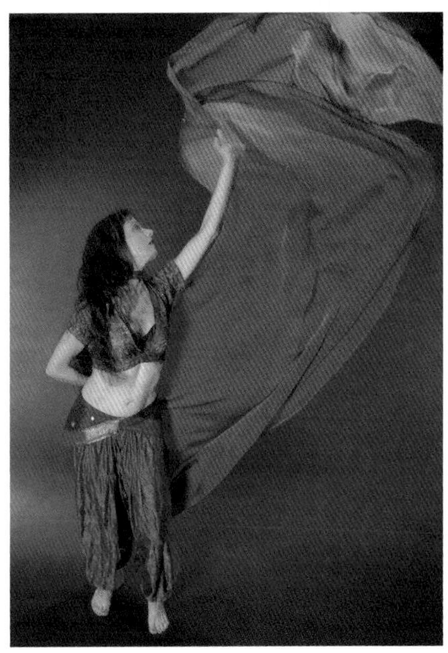

CASCADING LEFT AND RIGHT

Standing with the fabric behind you, drop your arms to your sides and extend them backward. Swing them together left and right. As you reach the final swing to the right, raise your right arm and perform a single lift and cascade. Your left arm should remain behind you.

When the cascade is complete, begin swinging your arms again, but this time allow the final swing to lead into a lift and cascade on your left side. As a last step, cut out the in-between swings and just perform left and right cascades one after the other.

MAKING THE VEIL DANCE

Beautiful veil work often comes from your own inspiration, rather than in formalized steps. These next few movements focus on providing you with a core of veil steps, while allowing you the freedom to experiment with the veil as an extension of your body.

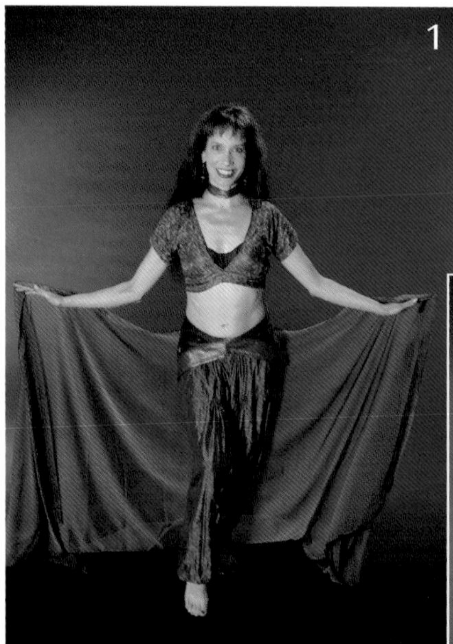

VEIL SWITCH

1 One of the most elegant movements, this is also one of the simplest. The step moves the veil gracefully around the body without looking jerky or awkward. The step requires eight counts. Begin in the veil foundation position.

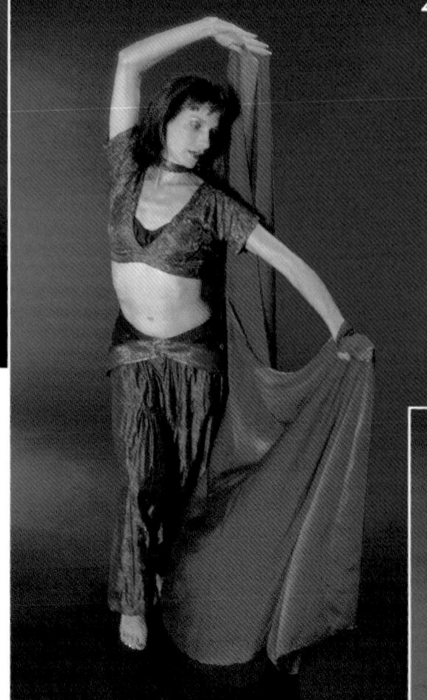

2 Raise your right arm and circle it around behind you, moving it clockwise and over your head for two counts.

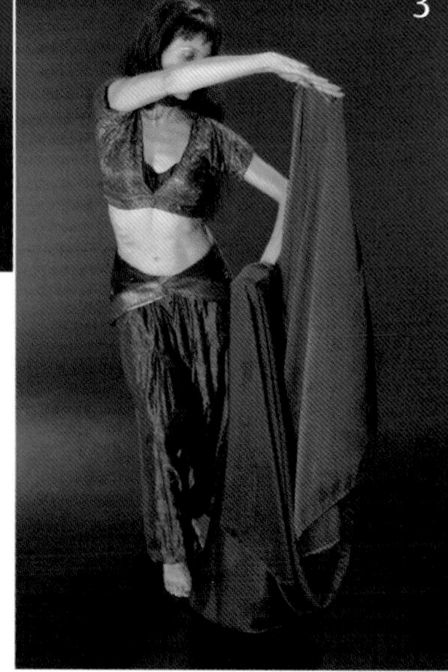

3 When your right arm begins to reach the front of your body, bend your left elbow, bringing your hand closer to your abdomen. Continue to move your right arm past your left until it sweeps fully to the front for one count.

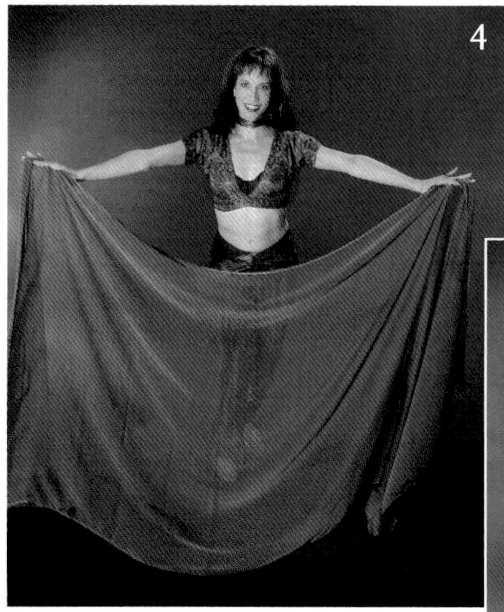

4 Hold both arms out again until they are back in their original position, with the exception that the veil is now in front of you. This is also one count.

5 With your left arm, bring the veil across the front of your body to the right. As your left arm passes your right arm, lead your right hand through the gap in the veil to pass to the left for one count.

6 Continue moving your left arm over and round your head until the veil is behind you for one count.

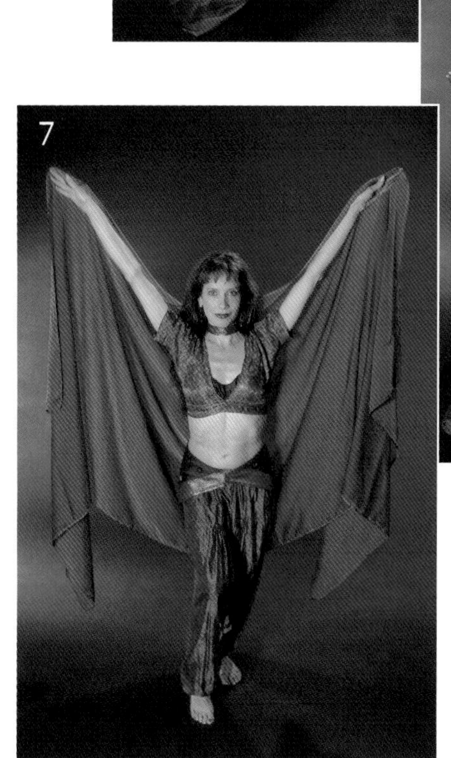

7 Return your left arm to its original position and slowly raise both arms above your head to finish. Let this section of the step comprise the final two counts.

PRACTICE

Repeat the right veil switch, then the left veil switch, four times each. Return to a right veil switch and perform one for eight counts, then four, then two. Repeat on the left.

SPINNING THROUGH THE DOOR

Take a few moments to review the cross step turn (p.65), both left and right, before learning this step.

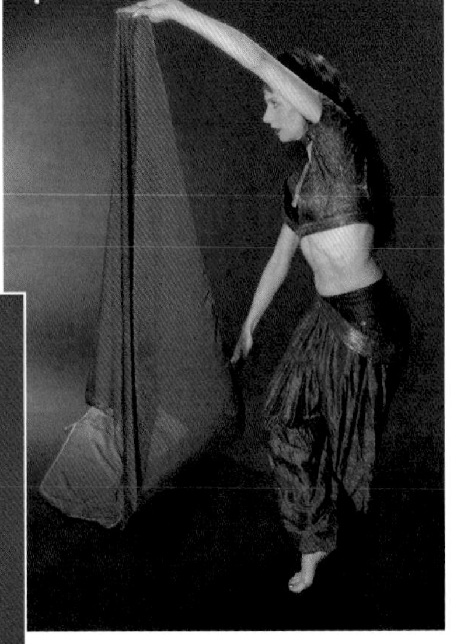

1 Raise your left arm and lower your right, holding the veil securely in both hands. Keeping your left arm high, sweep your right arm under and inside your left, while beginning a left cross step turn for two counts.

2 Begin to pivot on both feet and arch your back gently. As you spin round to face the back of your dancing space, your left arm should remain aloft as the right arm begins to arc in a wide circular upward swing. This also takes two counts.

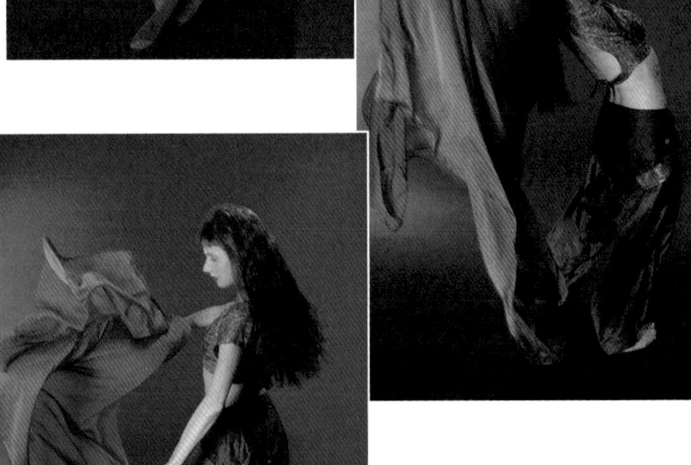

3 Continuing the turn without breaking the momentum for another two counts, sweep your left arm down and behind you, also in a wide circular arc. Quickly follow your left arm with your right while completing the pivot around to face front.

4 For the final two counts, as your left arm begins to swing back up to waist level during the completion of the turn, sweep your right arm out and down, also to waist level, until both arms are level. Repeat in the other direction.

PRACTICE

Start in a beautiful pose of your choosing and slowly switch the veil from left to right. Repeat twice, then change direction for another two switches. Finish with spinning through the door, once to the left and once to the right.

KISSING THE AUDIENCE

This is one step in which the dancer completely controls the veil's movements. The veil can be notoriously erratic and you never quite know if it's going to cooperate with you or not. But you can rely on this step to do what it is supposed to do if you perform the movements correctly.

1 Standing in a low foundation with the veil behind you, lean slightly forward. Leading with the upper sides of your arms and wrists, lift your arms up and forward, and cross them moderately in front.

2 Immediately flip the veil high up in front of you and out to your sides in a dramatic, V-shaped sweep.

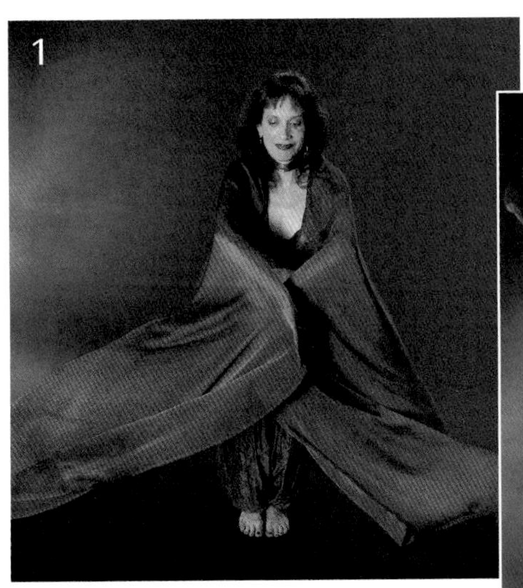

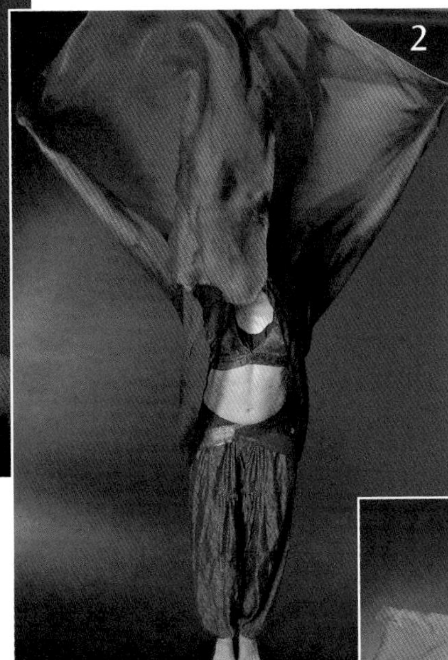

3 Without losing momentum, lower your arms by swinging them down and parallel in a large downward sweep, so that they almost meet in front of you.

PRACTICE

Repeat and experiment with speed to see what works best with your particular veil. This move should be done quickly and smoothly, but not so fast as to make the veil whippish. Because it is so beautiful, the kiss can be performed to each side as a whole set. So, a kiss front, turn to the left and kiss, then back and kiss, and lastly to the right and kiss. Smooches all around!

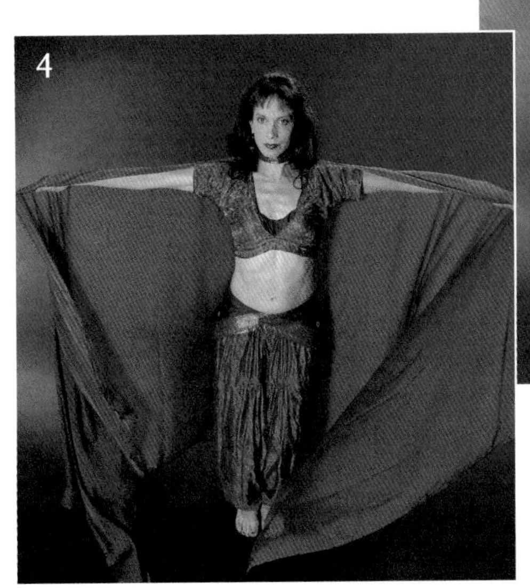

4 Follow through and complete the step by continuing the downward swing to thigh level. Finally swing your arms up and out to your sides, returning to the foundation position.

CREATING WINGS AND OFFERING VEIL

CREATING WINGS

1 Cascade the veil to the front and, with your arms extended diagonally away from your body, hold the veil draped over each thumb.

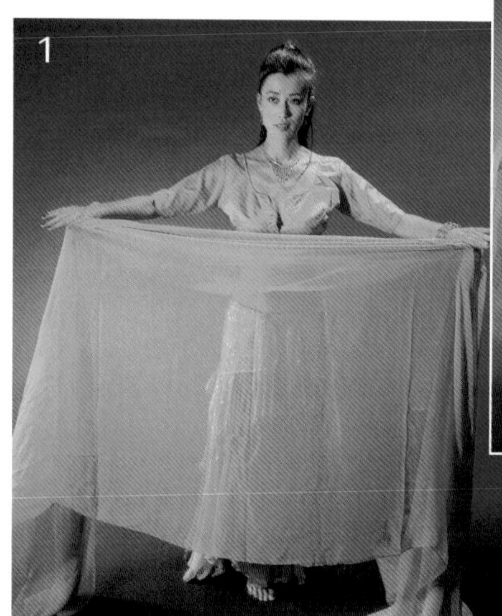

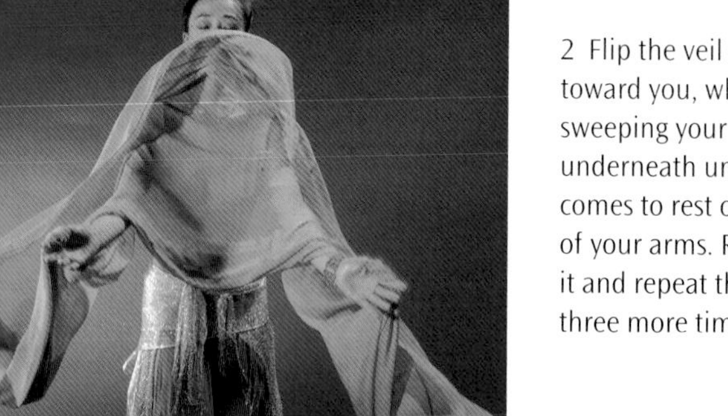

2 Flip the veil up and toward you, while sweeping your hands underneath until it comes to rest on top of your arms. Release it and repeat the flip three more times.

3 As you complete the last flip, gently extend your arms further out to your sides until the veil is taut. Hold the taut area against your neck while raising your arms high at the sides. Release. Now, in one quick, fluid movement, flip the veil, extend your arms and hit your neck with the taut veil edge. The veil will naturally collect itself at your neck as you raise your arms high at your sides. Release by tossing the veil down and gently forward in front of you.

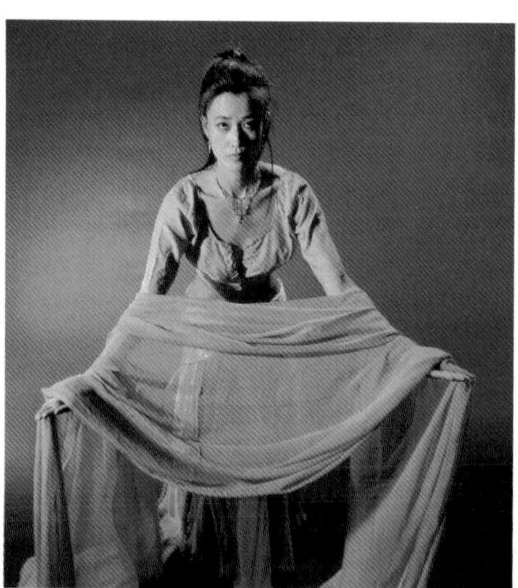

OFFERING VEIL

Although the offering veil is a separate step, it is also a nice way to close the creating wings veil. From the last wings position, bend your knees and lean forward. Gradually lower your arms and the veil will naturally slide down your chest and come to rest on your forearms. Begin slow, forward snake arms until the veil moves to rest across your wrists. Grasp the veil with your thumbs and sweep your arms underneath, flipping the veil forward and down. Cascade the veil back to rest behind you and return to foundation.

ANDROMEDA VEIL

When Andromeda's mother boasted that her daughter was more beautiful than the sea nymphs, they exacted revenge by pressuring Poseidon to release a sea monster to ravage the people of the land. The only way to stop the rampage was to sacrifice Andromeda to the creature. Chained to a rock by the sea and whipped by the ocean and wind, she bravely awaited her fate but was saved by Perseus. This veil movement is named for her.

PREPARATION

From the offering veil position, raise your arms high in the air, but without holding the veil in both hands. Allow the veil to fall over your shoulders. Lower your arms to your sides and bow slightly.

1 Lean softly to the left and look at your left arm. Swing it outside and round the veil until the fabric is wrapped twice round your wrist, resembling a cuff. Hold your left arm steady and gracefully lean to the right. Swing your right arm round the veil until it also has a veil cuff.

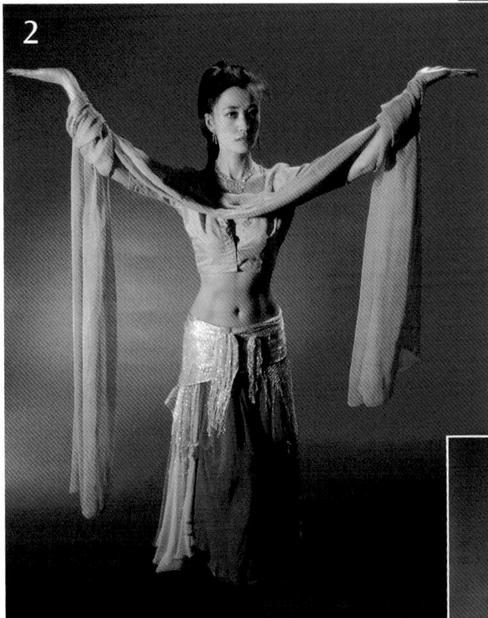

2 Raise both arms, now bound by veil chains, and sway back and forth, as though chained to a rock like Andromeda.

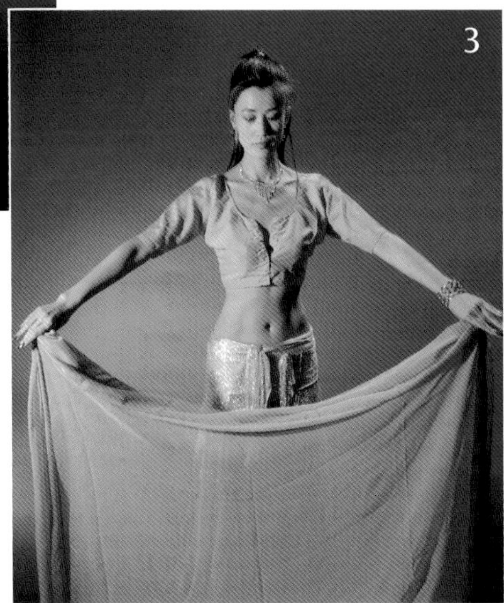

3 To release, lower your arms slowly while bending your knees and leaning forward. Slowly, using small circular movements, unwrap the veil from your arms. Lean further forward until gravity pulls the veil down to rest on your forearms and across your chest. Sweep your hands underneath and grasp the long side of the veil, flipping it over and straightening up. Cascade the veil back to rest behind you and return to foundation.

SANDSTORM VEIL

Complicated but visually stunning, the sandstorm is well worth learning. It is meant to be performed on the side of the body, to the left or right. As you master the movement, look in the mirror and you'll see the veil creating an amazing vortex like the eye of a sandstorm.

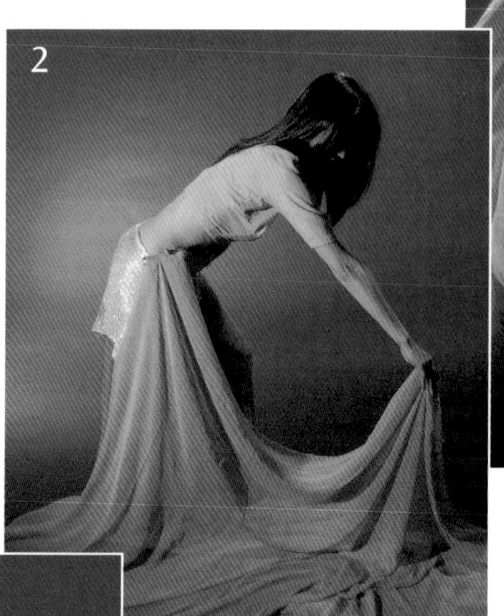

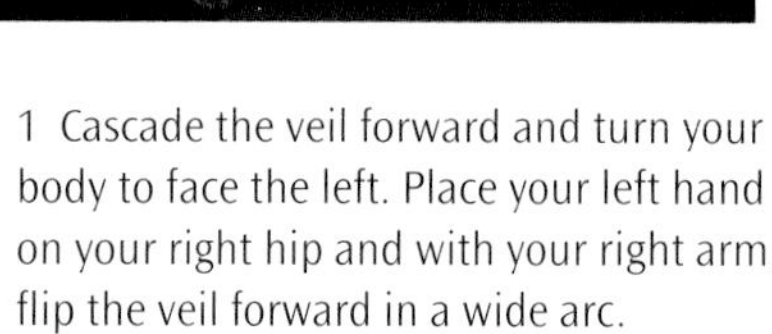

1 Cascade the veil forward and turn your body to face the left. Place your left hand on your right hip and with your right arm, flip the veil forward in a wide arc.

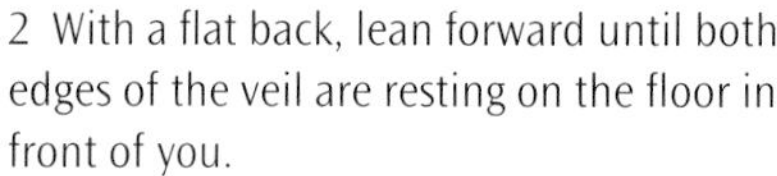

2 With a flat back, lean forward until both edges of the veil are resting on the floor in front of you.

3 Take your right arm and flip the veil back the same way you flipped it forward, in a high wide arc.

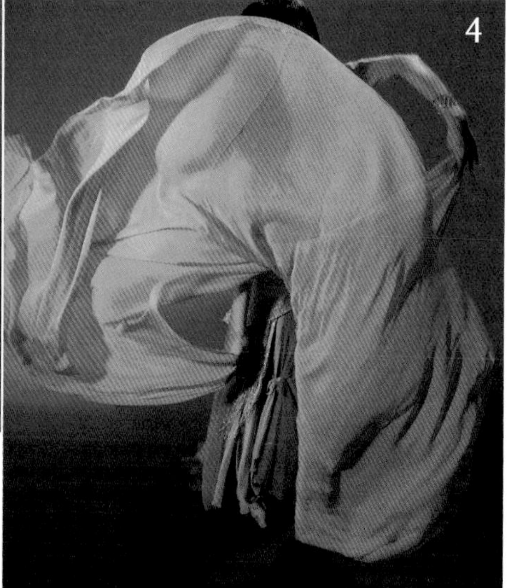

4 As your right arm passes your face, flip your left arm back, also sweeping in a high wide arc.

5 Continue moving your right arm in a full circle around the side of your body while following it with your left.

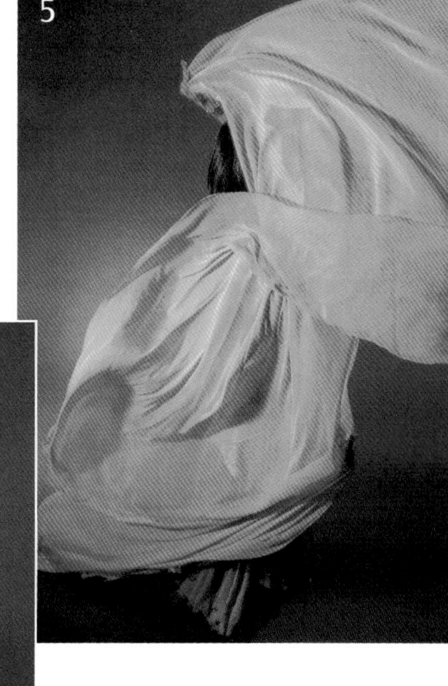

6 When your left arm is directly above your head, move to rest your hand on the back left side of your head.

7 Finish the right arm sweep by allowing it to pass once more over your head and down behind you. Flip the veil over your forearm. At this point your right arm will have completed one and a half circles.

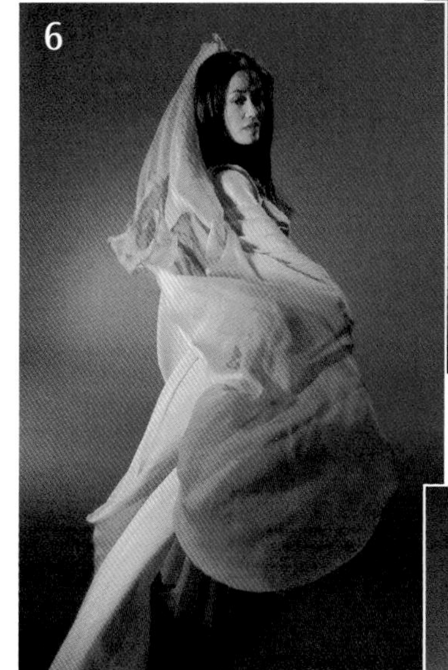

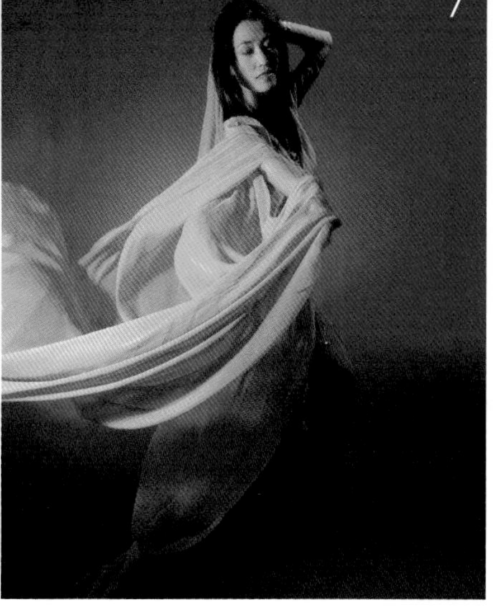

FINISHING TOUCHES
Here are two ways of completing the step. One is to reverse the storm until the veil is back in the start position. The other is called "sailing through the storm".

REVERSING THE STORM
Begin with your left arm. Sweep it in the opposite direction (forward and around) until the veil is no longer wrapped round it. Now simply sweep the veil forward in the same way it was swept back, following with your right arm until you are back in the starting position.

SAILING THROUGH THE STORM
Instead of flipping forward to release, hold the veil firmly in your left hand, which is resting on your head, and grasp the other end gently with your right thumb. Lift your right arm high into the air and begin spinning to the right, creating a large sail billowing behind you. To release, gradually slow to a halt and with both hands flip the veil forward to the ground, leaning with it. Cascade the veil back and return to veil foundation.

PRACTICE
Perform three complete sets of sandstorm veil, then try it on the other side. For a final step, move into sailing through the storm right after each sandstorm.

USING THE VEIL AS AN ACCENT

As well as being an extension of the body of the dancer, the veil can also act as a subtle accent to the movements, adding interest and drama to relatively simple steps.

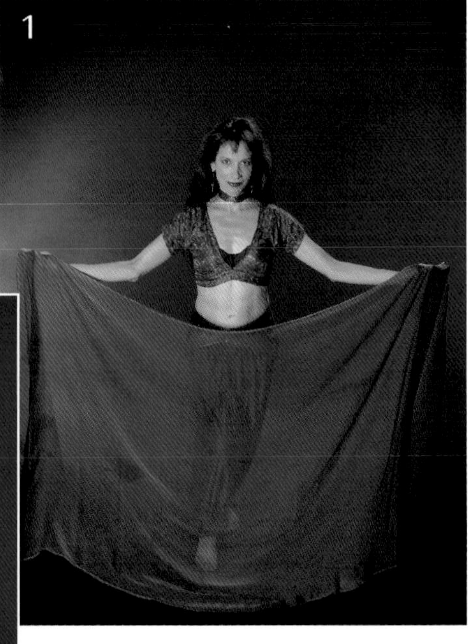

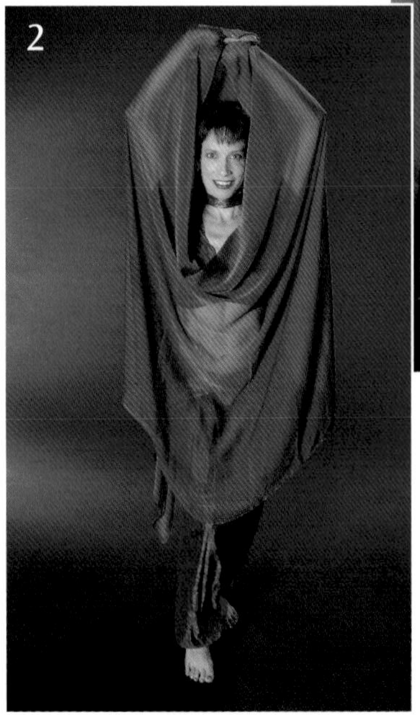

PRINCESS VEIL FRONT FACE FRAME

1 Cascade the veil in front of you and turn your hands until your palms are facing the ceiling.

2 Raise your arms up and bend them at the elbows. Rotate your hands out and round to the back so they meet at the top of your head, fingertips touching.

BACK FACE FRAME

Holding the veil behind you, raise your arms. Bending at the elbows, lean slightly back and touch your hands together over your head in the prayer position (right).

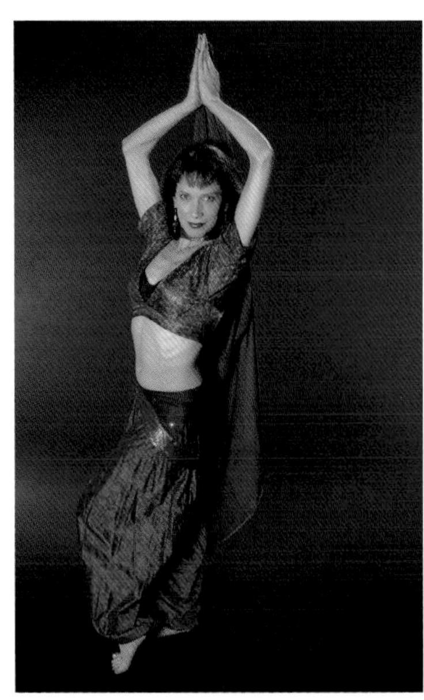

DANCING WITH THE FACE FRAME

When the veil frames your face to the front, most of your body is covered. The cobra neck slither (p.48) works perfectly because it is an interesting move in itself and loses nothing but gains everything by being framed. With the back face frame, the entire body is exposed. The cobra neck slither is again an excellent choice, as are hip drops (p.28) and hip rolls (p.32).

STEPPING OVER THE CURTAIN

1 Begin with a slow front cascade. With as much drama as you can muster, drop your body gently toward the front as the cascade rolls forward.

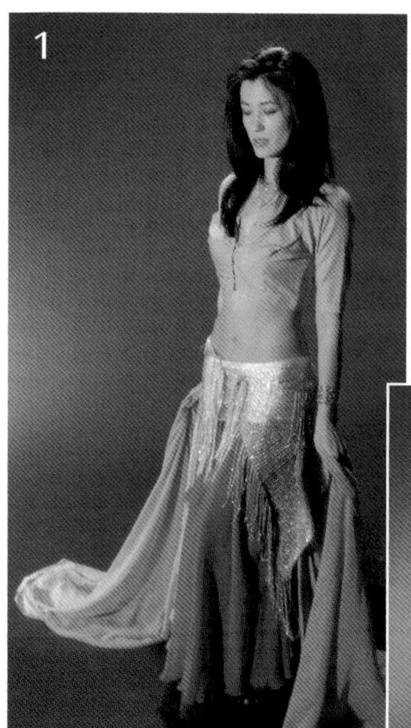

2 Guide the veil down and in, so that it hits your ankles and gathers there. Come up and dramatically flip your hair out of your face with an arched back.

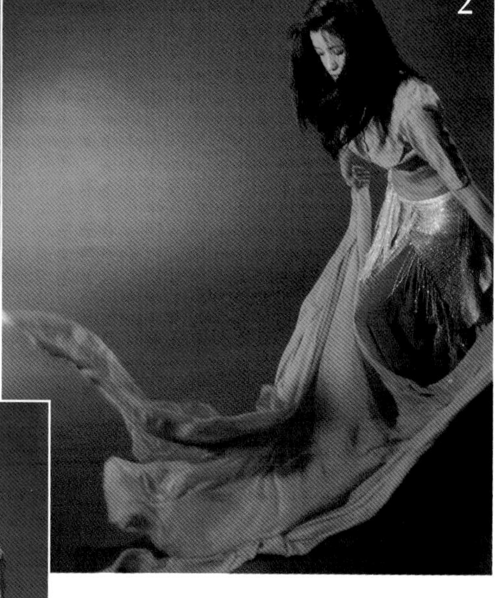

3 Slowly straighten your spine and rise up a little. Carefully and sensuously step over the veil with your left foot. Place your foot firmly on the floor and shift all your weight onto it. Pause for a count.

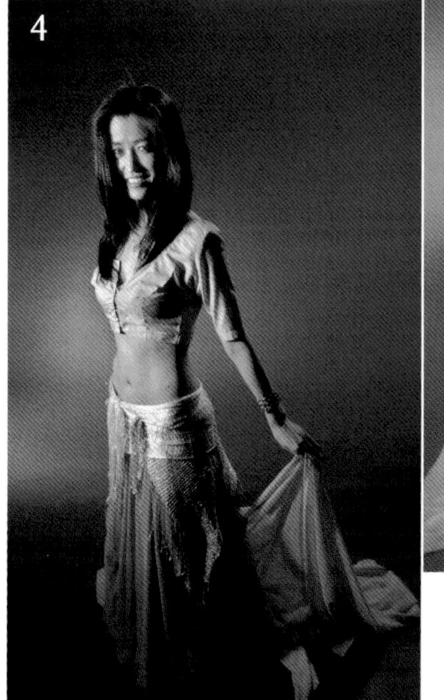

4 Complete the step by following with your right foot so the veil is completely behind you.

When using this technique, less is more. Only do this accent once in a dance, otherwise it can look as if you're skipping rope. It can be followed by other movements, such as body glimpsing (p.73), lift and cascade (p.80) or veil switch (p.82).

THE BUTTERFLY

The butterfly is tricky and takes some coordination, so be patient. Thinking carefully about how your arms move will help you to perform the step correctly.

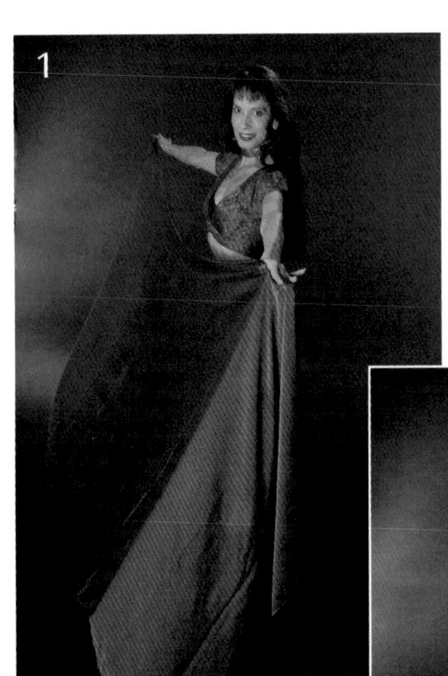

1 Cascade the veil to the front.

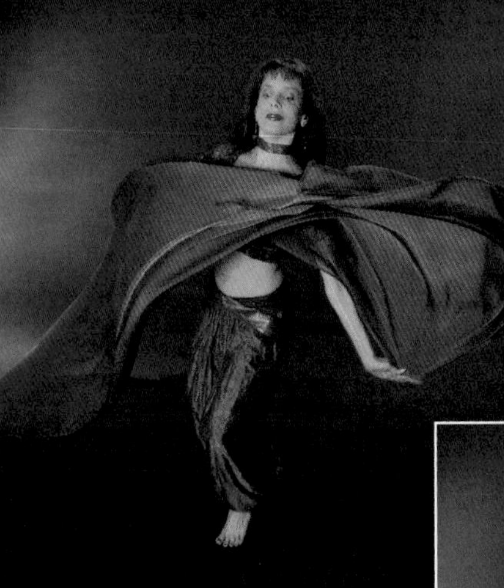

2 Sweep your left arm under the veil, bringing it up to chest level.

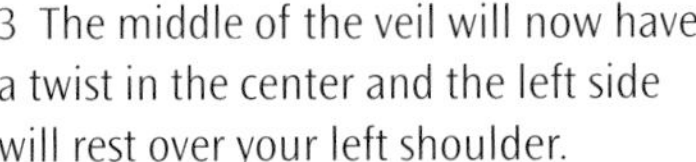

3 The middle of the veil will now have a twist in the center and the left side will rest over your left shoulder.

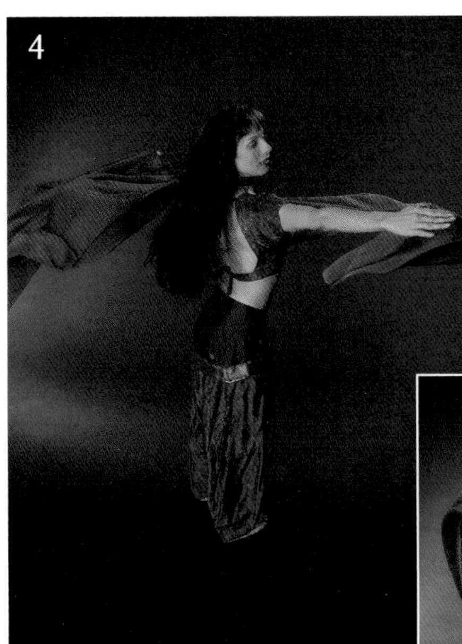

4 Begin turning to the right and stop quickly when you come around to the front after the second rotation.

5 Gently dip low by bending your knees. At the same time, sweep your right arm down, forward and up, while sweeping your left arm down, back and up.

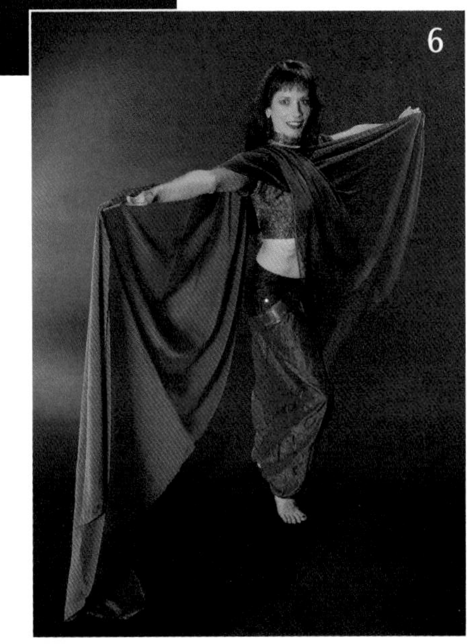

6 The veil will still have a twist in the middle, but it will now rest over your right shoulder. Begin turning again, this time toward the left. After the second rotation, stop again in the center. Dip low and swing your right arm down and back while sweeping your left arm down, forward, then up. The veil will now be resting back on your left shoulder. Start spinning again and switch after the second rotation. Release by unflipping the veil from whichever arm it is resting on in your final turn.

PRACTICE

It's best to follow this complex, fast-moving step with something simple and slow. Perform three full butterflies. After the release (step 6), perform a half veil switch (p.82) or a cascade (p.80) to position the veil behind you.

THE ENVELOPE

Deeply mysterious and sensuous, the envelope walks the fine line between suggestion and seduction because of its method of final unveiling. Temper this by adding a sense of playfulness and character to the earlier steps.

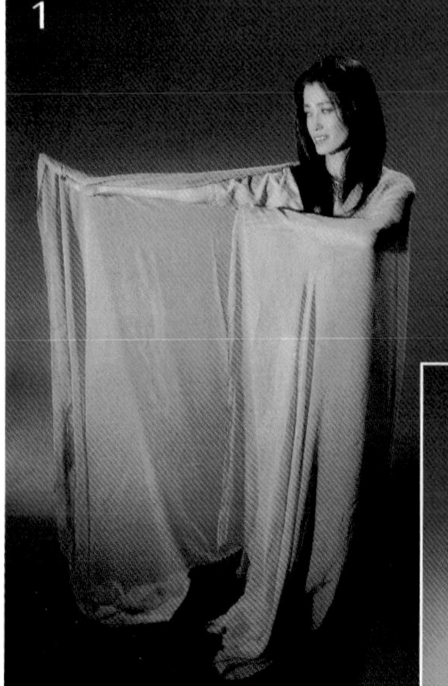

1 The envelope should always start mid-spin. This distracts the audience and prevents them from predicting what will happen next. Start spinning in whichever direction you feel most comfortable and raise your arms to shoulder level.

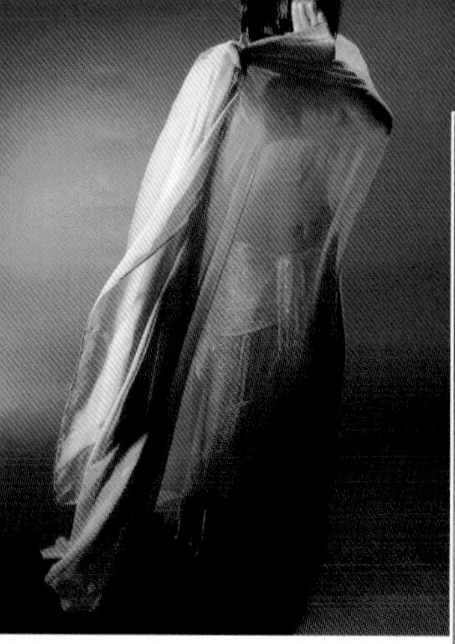

2 As you turn, bring your arms and hands together until they meet in the center. Grab both ends of the veil in your right hand, releasing the left. Push gently against the veil with your left hand to pull it taut.

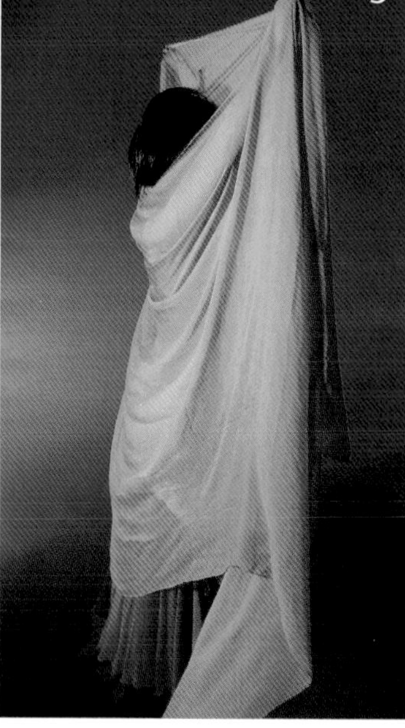

3 Lift the veil over your head until you are completely surrounded by the material. It may catch on your hair on the way up, but don't let that interrupt you. Your hair will eventually fall inside and rest back where is supposed to.

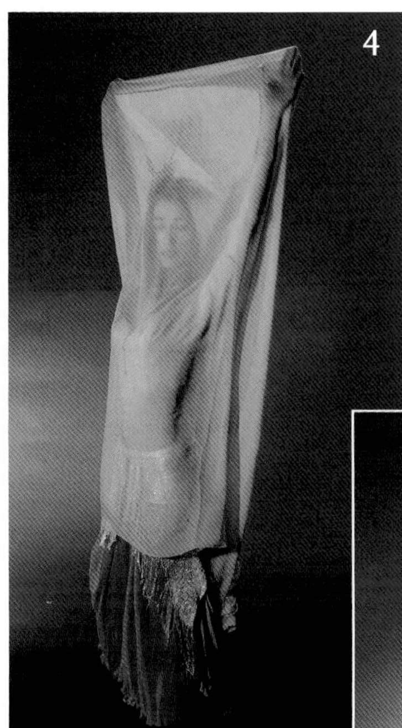

4 Gradually stop spinning and begin some of your favourite dance movements. You can face to the front or diagonally, depending on the movement you choose. For example, hip rolls (p.32), chest circles (p.45) and shimmies (p.38) should be performed facing front. Hip drops (p.28) and undulations (p.42) should be done on the diagonal for maximum effect.

5 While dancing some hip-focused movements, spread the opening of the veil at the top by separating your thumb and forefinger. Look up and lower the veil down over your head until it is in front of your eyes.

Bring the veil forward so that you can see out of it. Here's a chance to use facial expressions to convey emotions. A fun idea to try is to peer out of the veil meaningfully, looking left to right as if you're searching for someone. Get someone's attention and give a playful wink.

6 Wrap your arms behind your head, placing your hands almost on top of your crown, creating a mask effect with the veil. Very deep and low hip rolls work well for this part of the envelope. Finish this mischief by spinning again, just two rotations, and lifting the veil back up above you.

FINISHING THE ENVELOPE

7 Finishing the envelope and releasing the veil is a delight because the exit is as beautiful as the entrance. With the veil above your head, allow your left hand to peek out at the top and begin snaking it down.

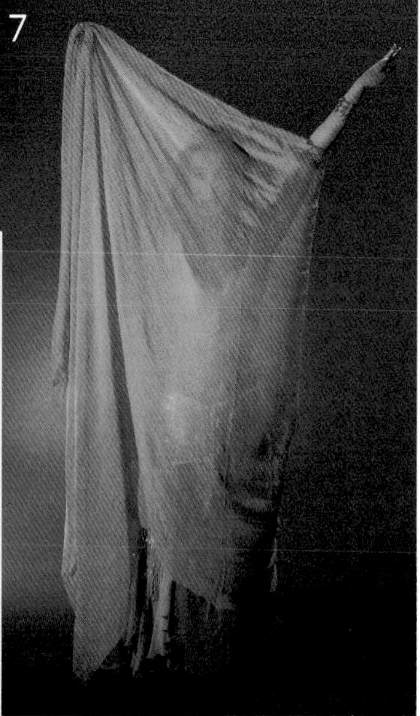

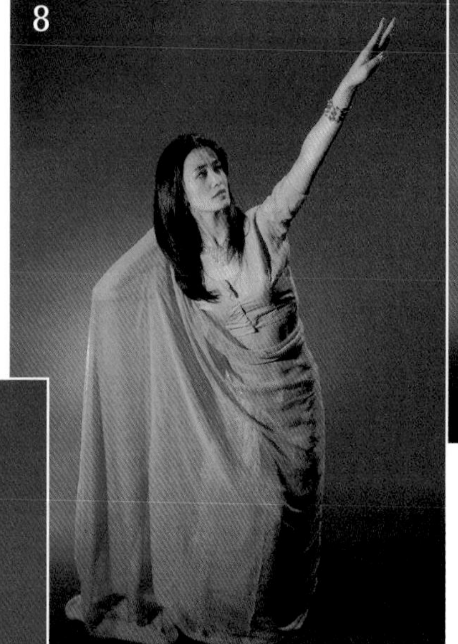

8 Slowly lower your right arm while extending the snaking motion down your left. As your right arm continues its descent, allow your head to come out and follow it with your chest. When your upper body begins to be exposed, movements such as chest circles (p.45) or undulations (p.42) are a great way to slide out of the envelope.

9 When your entire body down to your hips is out of the envelope, finish in one fluid motion. Turn round to the back, grab the left side of the veil with your free (left) hand so you have one end in each hand.

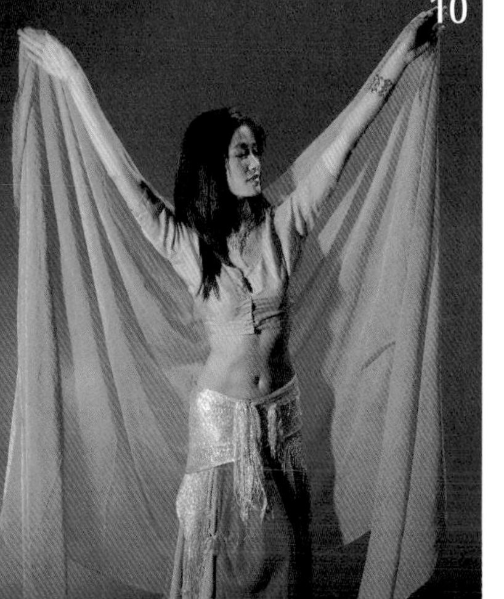

10 Turn to face front. With a flourish, separate the veil ends for a full body view until your arms are raised high behind you. Slowly lower them back down to the veil foundation position.

SPINNING BARREL TURN

All the turns and spinning techniques taught earlier can be accented with veil work. The three-point (p.66), dervish (p.68) and cross step (p.65) turns are fast enough to gather air and lift the veil so it surrounds you like a gossamer mist. Using the veil's versatility, add this turn to your repertoire.

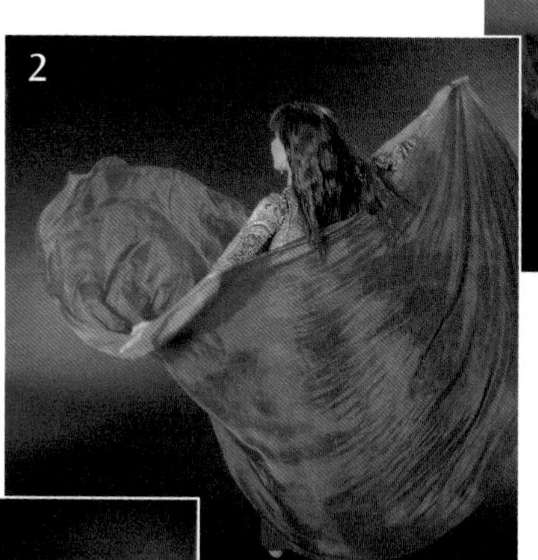

1 Begin by spinning slowly to the right, making small steps. As your body begins its second turn, drop your right arm in a circular sweep downward and raise your left arm in a circular sweep upward.

2 Without breaking the momentum, sweep your right arm up and your left arm down as your body continues turning to face the back of your dance space.

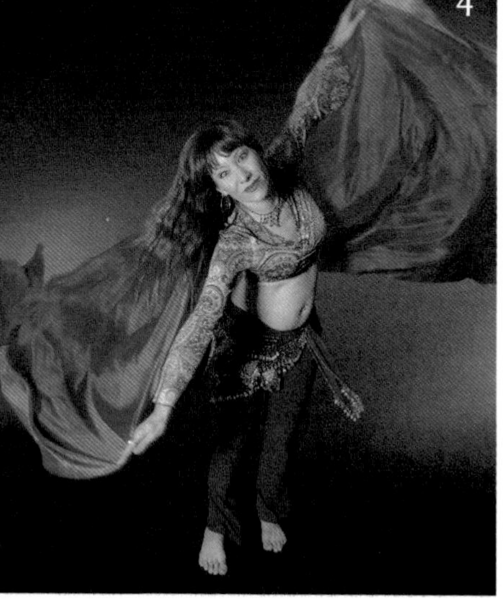

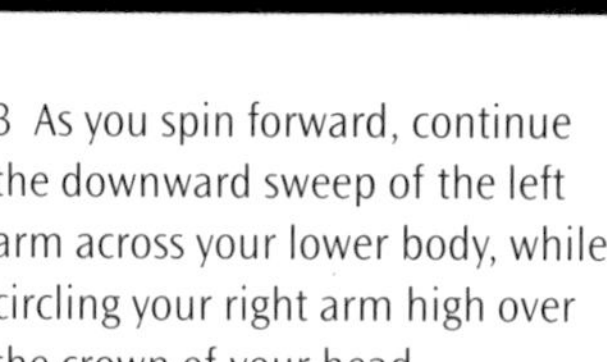

3 As you spin forward, continue the downward sweep of the left arm across your lower body, while circling your right arm high over the crown of your head.

4 Keep spinning and circling your arms while gaining in speed. The veil will flow round you, creating an almost uninterrupted halo of fabric, similar to a rolling barrel.

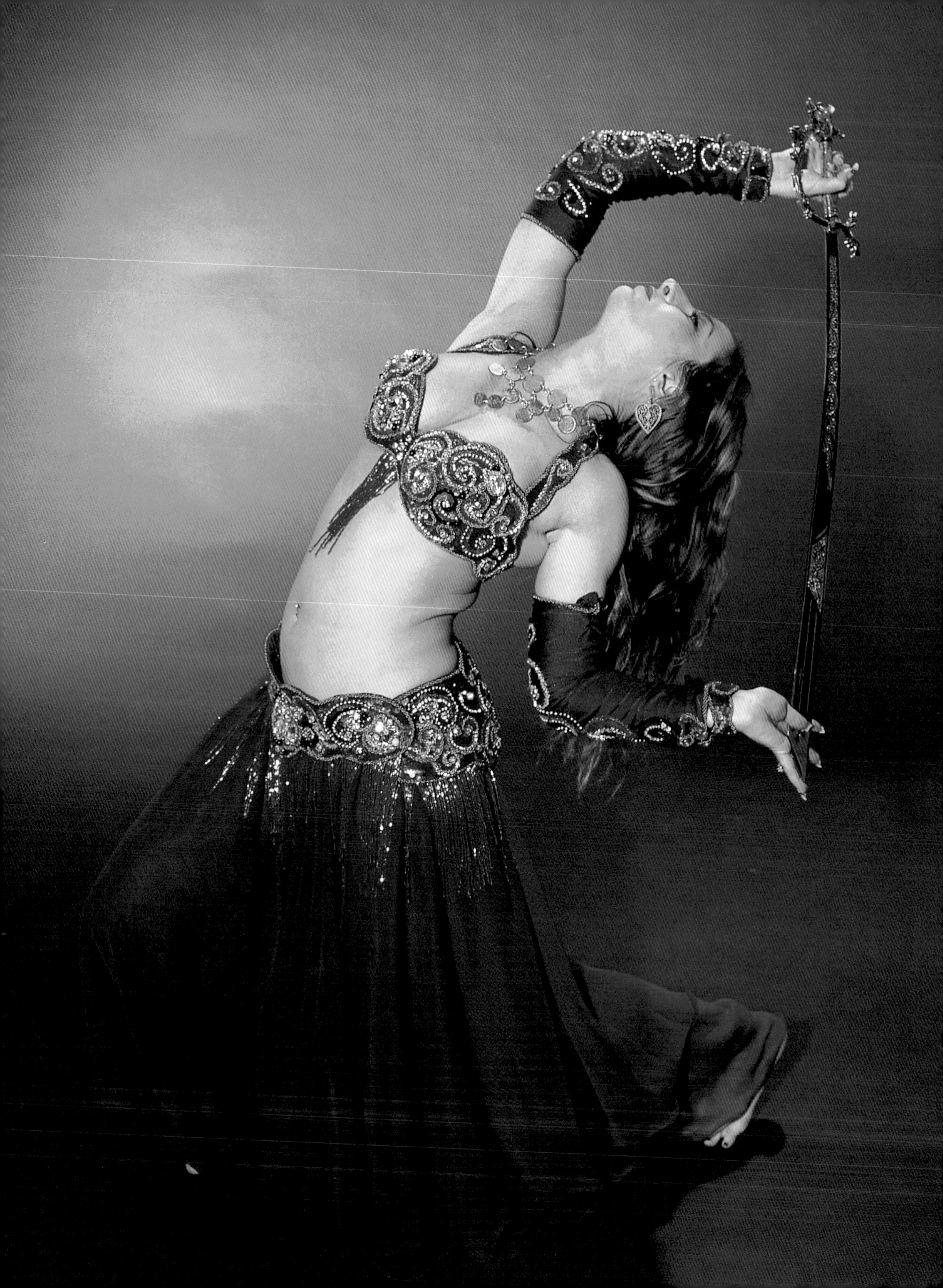

5 Drawing on power

Sword dancing embodies the warrior goddess in every woman. It empowers a dancer and allows her to extend her vision to include incredible images of power, freedom, risk, danger and mystery. As you learn to dance with a sword, always take your time and go slowly. The sword dance is so stunning, compelling and magical that there is never any need to rush it. Move carefully and deliberately, instilling feeling and heart into each step, and the routine will do the rest!

Beginners should start with a very dull practice sword and handle it with great care to avoid injury. Most practice swords are made of lightweight compressed aluminum or layered tin, with a thin simple handle and covered scabbard. The blade itself is gently curved and usually two sided, meaning that there is a cutting edge running across the bottom as well as the first few inches of the top. A practice sword will have only one point at the tip, with the blade and the point filed very dull to minimize injury if an accident or slip should occur.

Professional swords are extremely beautiful and sophisticated but can cause injury if mishandled. I advise my students not to pick up a professional sword until they have mastered the dance with a practice one. A rule of thumb is when you are completely comfortable with your practice sword and can get through the entire sword lesson four times back to back without losing the sword even once, you can consider taking the leap to the professional sword.

The most common professional sword is the scimitar. Forged out of heavy steel and weighing about 2kg (4½lb), the scimitar's blade is usually about 1m (3ft 3in) long. It has a single curved cutting edge and boasts a very ornate handle that counterbalances the weight of the blade.

HOLDING THE SWORD

Remember that even a dull sword is still a weapon and should be held like one, with respect and delicacy. Always hold the handle of the sword with your dominant hand – the hand you write with. Grasp the sword in front of you with the blade facing the ceiling, gripping the handle firmly with your entire fist. Open your other hand into the offering position and rest the blade of the sword delicately on your first two fingers. Don't ever grab and hold the blade with a full hand or fist. From this position, lift the blade up in front of you and take a close look at it. If there is a sharp edge on the top and the bottom, then it is a double-edged sword. In that case, lightly slide your fingers toward the handle until they are past the second blade. If there is no second blade, then wherever your hand most feels comfortable is perfect.

PLACING THE SWORD ON YOUR HEAD

The practice sword must be extremely blunt. Swords do fall off, especially at first, so it is essential to practice your disaster recovery techniques before you start learning to sword dance.

PREPARATION

In order to learn without fear, you must love your sword. Hold the sword in your hands. Run your fingers across the blade and grasp it tightly in both hands to learn where it can be caught so it doesn't injure you. Toss it up and down gently and catch it with both hands. Once you are comfortable with your sword, you will know how to prevent disasters or repair them with dignity.

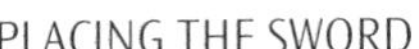

PLACING THE SWORD

1 Hold the sword out in front of you at a level just below your hips. Grasping the handle with one hand and supporting the blade with two fingers of the other hand, begin making large undulations.

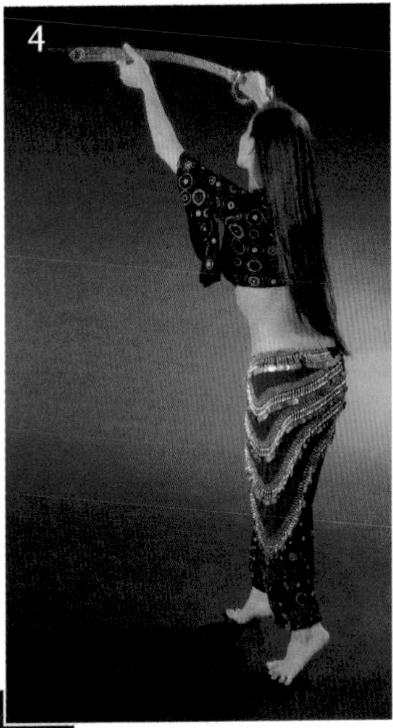

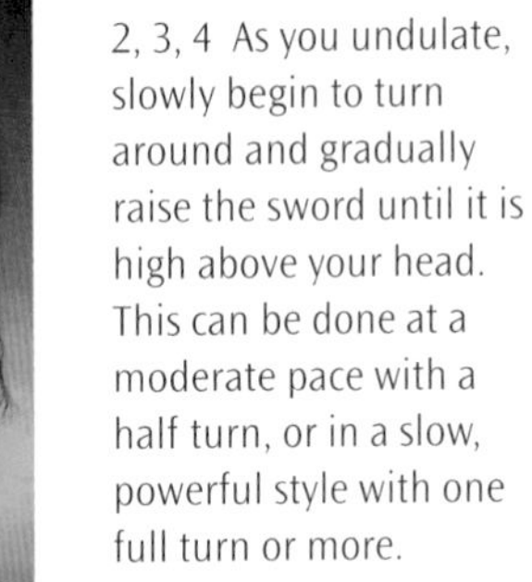

2, 3, 4 As you undulate, slowly begin to turn around and gradually raise the sword until it is high above your head. This can be done at a moderate pace with a half turn, or in a slow, powerful style with one full turn or more.

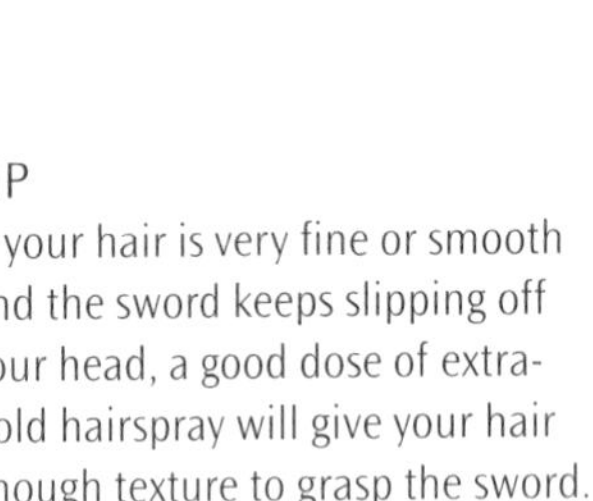

TIP

If your hair is very fine or smooth and the sword keeps slipping off your head, a good dose of extra-hold hairspray will give your hair enough texture to grasp the sword.

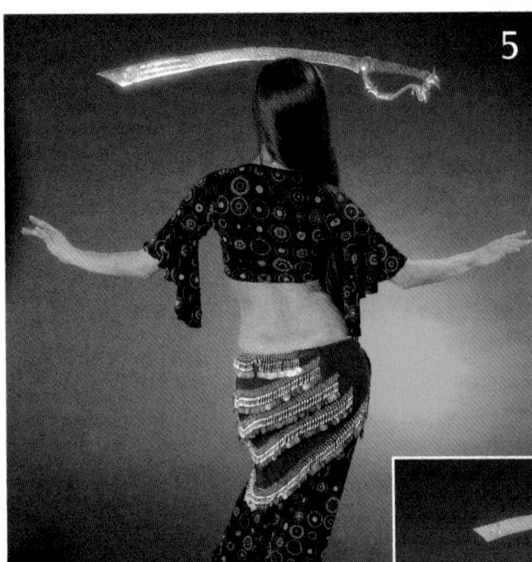

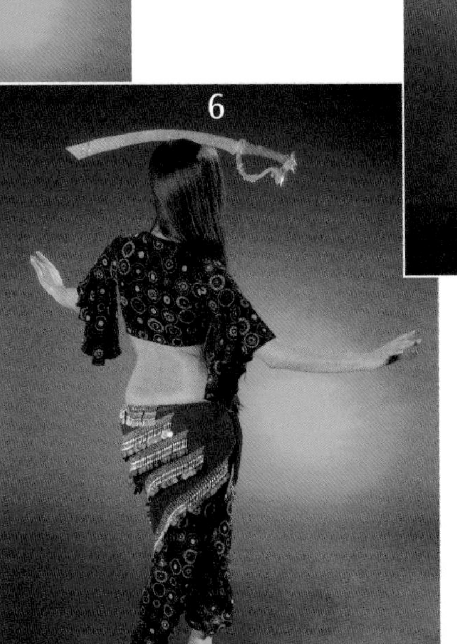

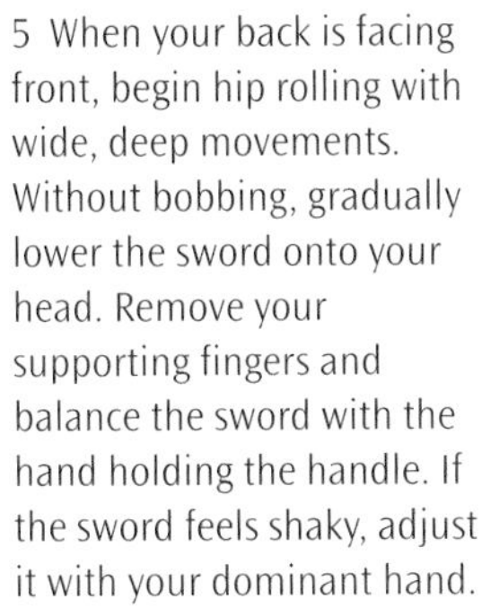

5 When your back is facing front, begin hip rolling with wide, deep movements. Without bobbing, gradually lower the sword onto your head. Remove your supporting fingers and balance the sword with the hand holding the handle. If the sword feels shaky, adjust it with your dominant hand.

6 Gradually stop hip rolling. Lift your left foot up and over your right, placing the ball of your foot firmly on the floor next to your right foot.

7 Pivot on your feet slowly so as not to knock the sword off-balance and turn around to face front again.

PRACTICE

Try snake arms (p.54), hip drops (p.28) , hip thrusts (p.31), hip rolls (p.32), basic walking (p.58) and undulations (p.42), all with the sword in place.

The key to good sword work is to make sure your head doesn't bob up and down – if it does, the sword will slide off. Look in the mirror and find a point behind you that you can use as a mark. It should be exactly at the middle of the blade. This small spot is your "bob" mark. By focusing on this spot, you'll be able to see if you are bobbing and correct yourself. To prevent bobbing, bend your knees a little more than usual to increase the movement range.

ADJUSTING THE SWORD

If you feel the sword starting to slip, reach up with your dominant hand, grasp the handle and gently readjust the sword's position. If the sword dips unevenly to the left, slide it to the right and vice versa.

TAKE CARE

Always be aware of safety. If the sword has slipped beyond a point where it can be adjusted or caught, then hop out of the way and let it drop. It will make a clang, but no harm will be done. Your dainty little toes are much more important than a piece of metal.

FLOOR WORK

Boasting a Hollywood level of drama and sensuality, floor work with the sword demands considerable skill and grace on the part of the dancer. Start by learning the body movements without the sword. When you've memorized them thoroughly, add the sword.

PREPARATION: DESCENDING TO THE FLOOR

With the sword on your head, place 80 percent of your weight on your left leg. Slide your right leg forward, around and behind you in a large wide circle. Slide your left leg forward into a deep lunge until your right knee touches the floor. Transfer 80 percent of your body weight onto your right knee by leaning back until you are in a full kneel. Slide your left foot forward until your leg is completely extended. Then sweep your left leg around to the back and drag it forward until it is parallel with your right leg and you are kneeling on both knees. This step does take a lot of strength; if you cannot do it yet, just kneel down on both knees, one leg at a time. Keep practicing as best you can without hurting yourself and you will succeed when your muscles are stronger.

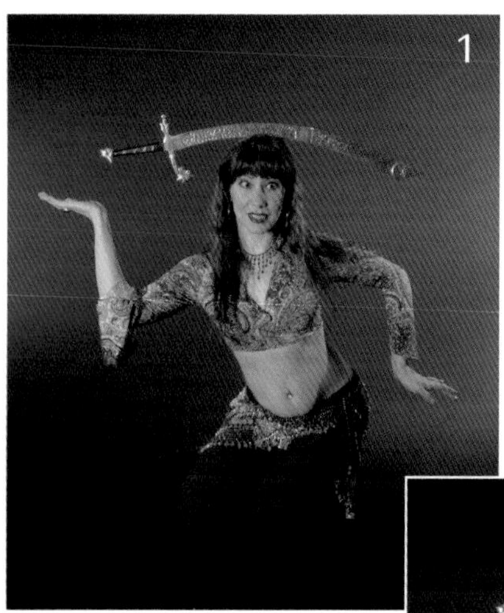

IN THE LAMP

1 While on your knees, hold your hands in front of you in prayer position. Begin to circle your hips around to the right. On the third circle, as your hip reaches the left side, push it out and down until you are almost sitting on your heels far over to the left. Place your arms in the genie position, with your left arm low and right arm high. Pause for a moment.

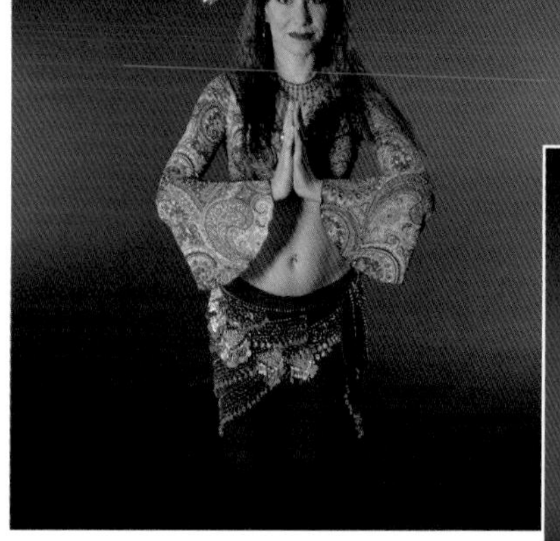

2 Resume the hip circle while lifting up and returning to center as your hips move to the right.

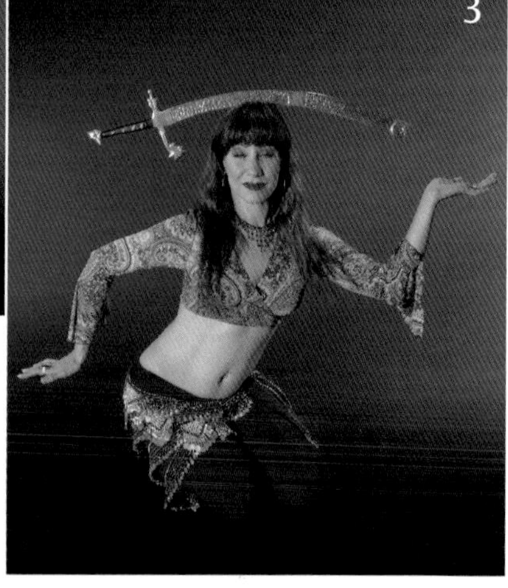

3 After two more hip circles, when your hip reaches the right side, push it out and down until you are almost sitting on your heels far to the right. This time, reverse the genie arm position, so your right hand is low and the left hand is high. Pause for a moment and lift up, returning to center while resuming your hip circle. Without breaking the hip circle, repeat the movement three more times on each side.

LAZY CROSS KICK

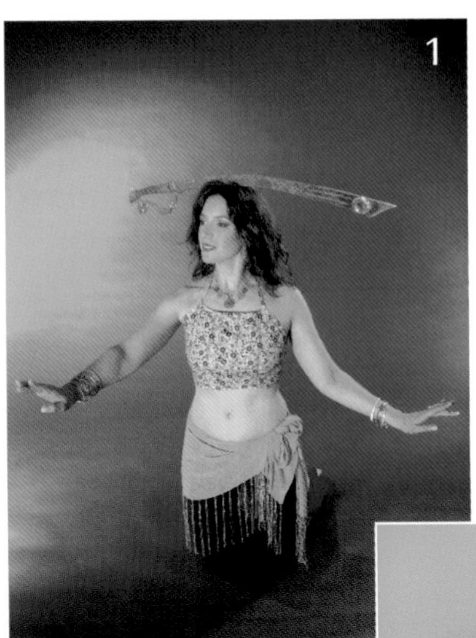

1 Begin by kneeling with your knees slightly apart and your arms in foundation with basic hands. Sit down on your heels, using the soles of your feet as a cushion for your bottom.

2 Reach your left arm behind you and lean diagonally back in that direction until your palm is flat on the floor. Bend your elbow, transferring your weight to your arm and away from your right leg.

PRACTICE

Despite its name, this step isn't so lazy. Don't be surprised if you have trouble keeping your leg up at first. Just keep at it and you will improve.

3 When free from pressure, extend your right leg straight out and lift it 10cm (4in) off the floor. With your free arm, reach over across your chest.

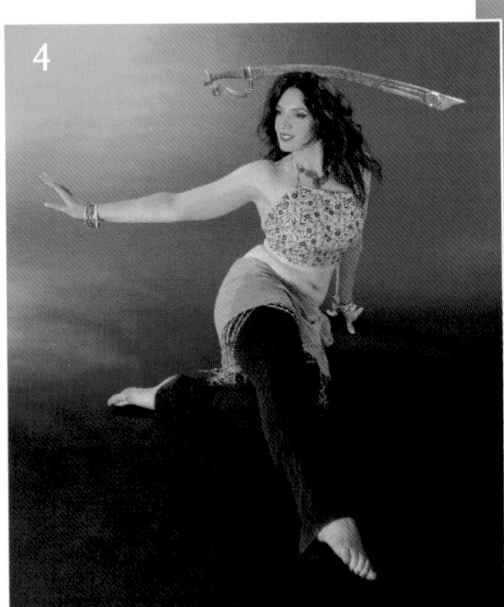

4 In one very slow continuous motion, swing your right leg across the floor all the way to your left side without dropping it, while swinging your right arm to the left side in a gentle gliding motion. Return your leg back to the left in the same way, simultaneously returning the arm to the right. Repeat the leg/arm cross twice more before coming out of the movement.

THE RESURRECTION

I always encourage my students to use creative visualization to add an extra layer of emotion to their developing skills. In order to perform this movement properly, think about the image you are trying to convey – the idea that a mummy, stiff and dead, is being resurrected and slowly coming alive. Another great visualization is to think of a caterpillar building a stiff cocoon round itself, then emerging as a beautiful butterfly. Remember to carry out this movement as slowly as you possibly can to promote the concept of metamorphosis.

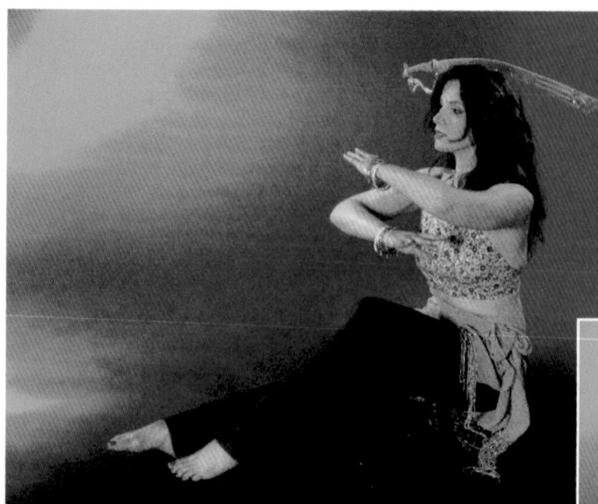

1 After descending to the floor, slowly sit back to the right of your heels. One by one, carefully swing your legs out in front of you and to the right, so that your left side is facing front. Keeping your spine very straight, hinge at the waist and lean forward, reaching for your feet. Cross your arms at the wrists and begin slow, sultry snake arms.

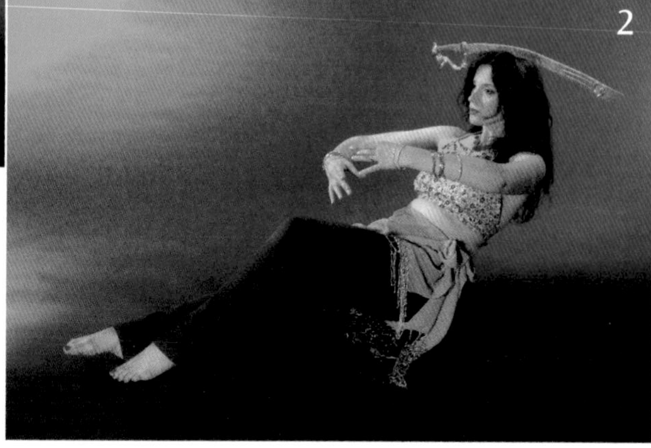

2 Curl your spine and begin to lean back, snaking your arms and hands up over your body. As your hands pass over each part of you (feet, calves, thighs, hips and so on), lock that part stiff. The idea is that you are mummifying yourself for eternity.

WARNING
You need to be very strong to perform this movement, so if you feel any strain in your lower spine or neck as you lean back, stop and don't go any further.

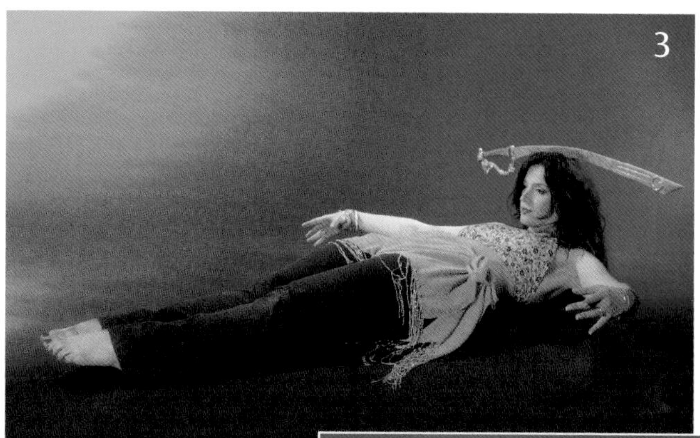

3 Keep snaking and leaning back until your shoulder blades rest on the floor. Keep your chin tucked firmly into your chest and your head elevated. Snake your arms out to the sides.

4 Slowly place your hands on the floor and swing them out to the sides until they are diagonally extended from each shoulder. Hold for a moment.

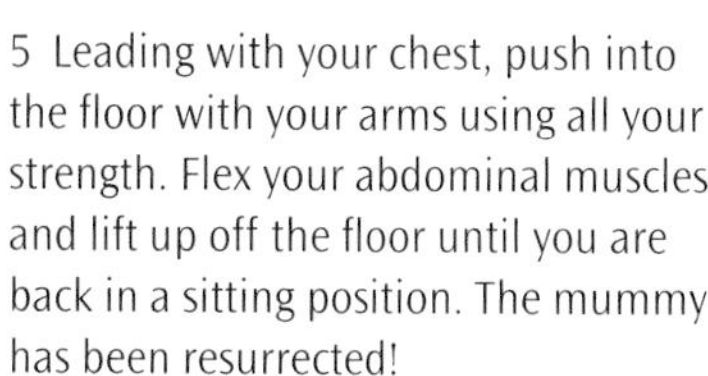

5 Leading with your chest, push into the floor with your arms using all your strength. Flex your abdominal muscles and lift up off the floor until you are back in a sitting position. The mummy has been resurrected!

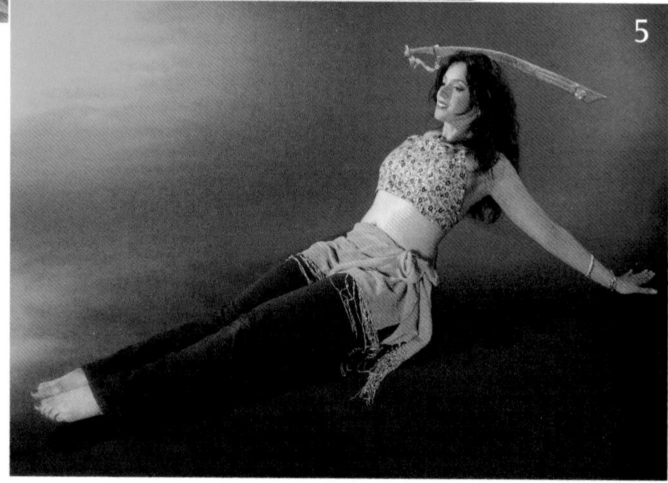

REMOVING THE SWORD

Even though, at this point, the essential elements of the sword routine are over, the removal of the sword should be as ceremonial as the placing of it on your head.

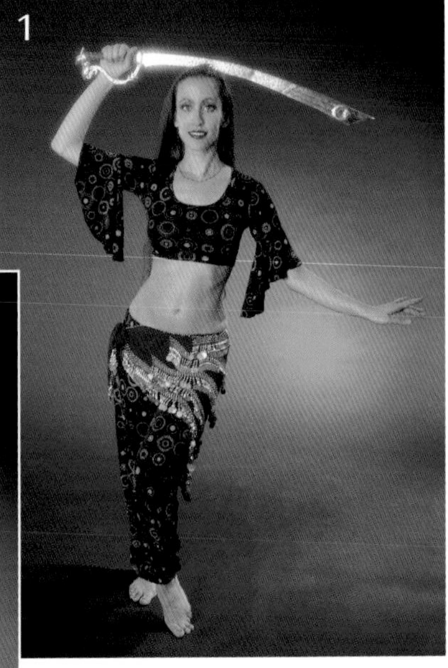

A SIMPLE METHOD

1 Leading with your elbow and then your wrist, raise your dominant arm up. When it is at shoulder level, extend your arm and turn it until your palm is facing up. Again leading with the wrist, bend your elbow and grasp the handle of the sword.

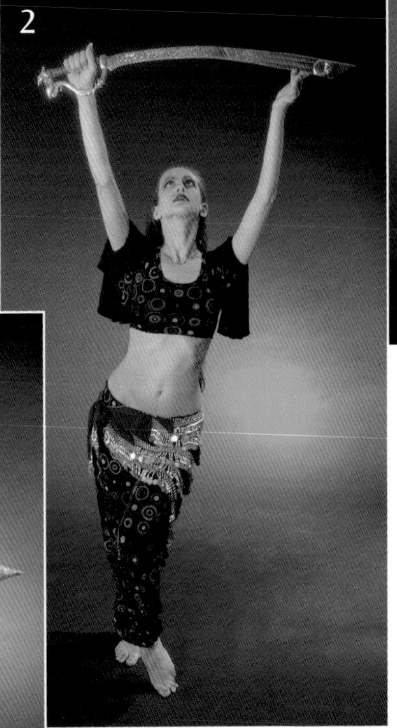

2 Carefully lift the sword straight off your head. Reach your free hand up to the blade so it rests gently on your fingertips. Without bending your elbows, lower the sword in front of you, following its descent with your eyes.

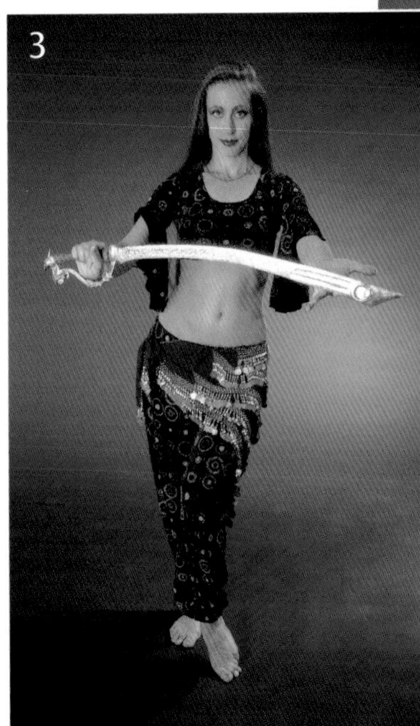

3 Stop lowering the sword when your arms are just above waist level, then move into a lovely pose of your choosing.

A FANCY OPTION

In this finale step, you remove the sword while spinning. Begin to turn and, using the method described in step 1, raise your dominant arm up and grasp the sword handle. Continue spinning and lift the sword straight up. Lower it in front of you, supporting the blade with two fingers of your other hand until it is at face level. Stop spinning and continue lowering the sword until your arms are at waist level. Move into a beautiful pose to finish the set.

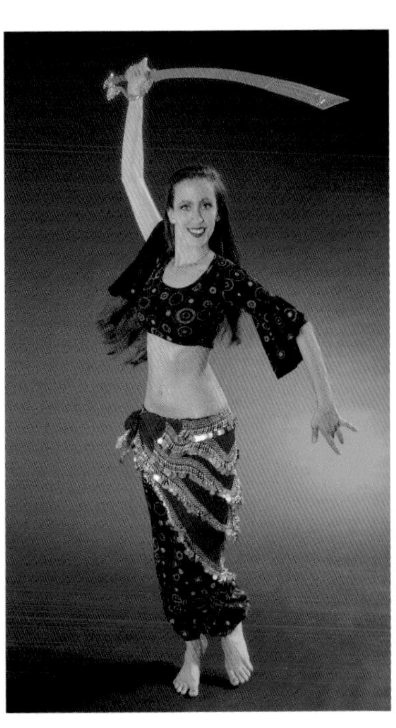

TRIPLE CIRCLE

At the climax of this movement, three parts of you will be circling: your arms, your body and your hips! The triple circle can be used before the sword is placed on your head or after it has been removed.

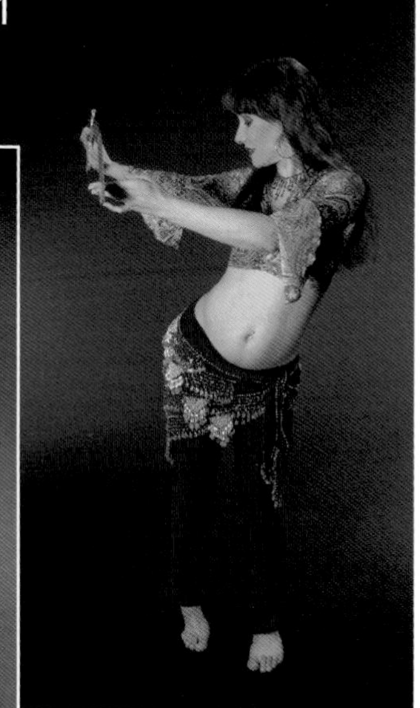

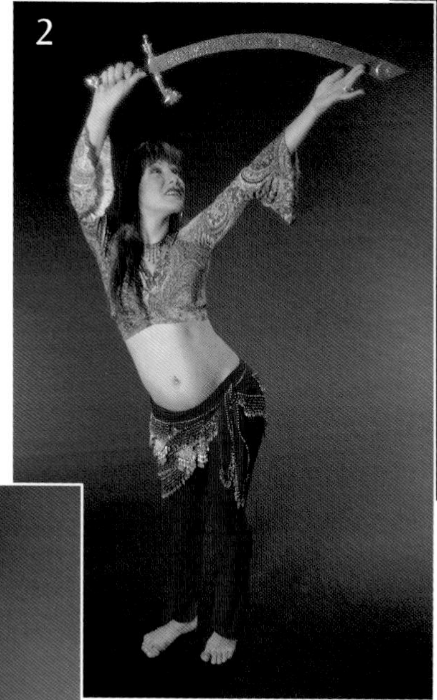

1 Holding the sword at chest level, hip roll (p.32) in wide circles, left and right. Make your circles as big and bold as you can.

2 Begin to draw a circle around your body with the sword by slowly raising it up while hip rolling, then bringing it over your head.

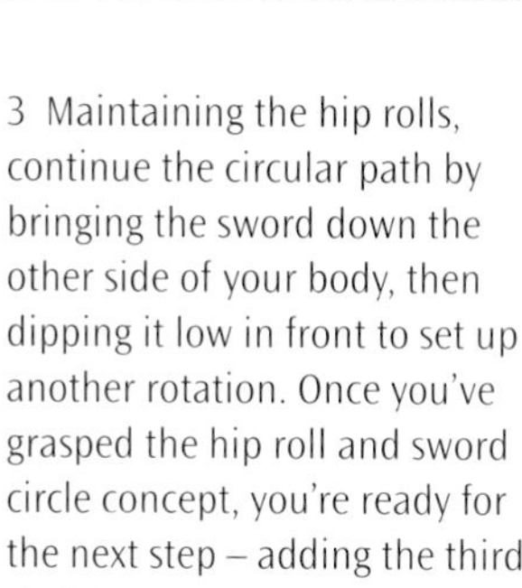

3 Maintaining the hip rolls, continue the circular path by bringing the sword down the other side of your body, then dipping it low in front to set up another rotation. Once you've grasped the hip roll and sword circle concept, you're ready for the next step – adding the third circle!

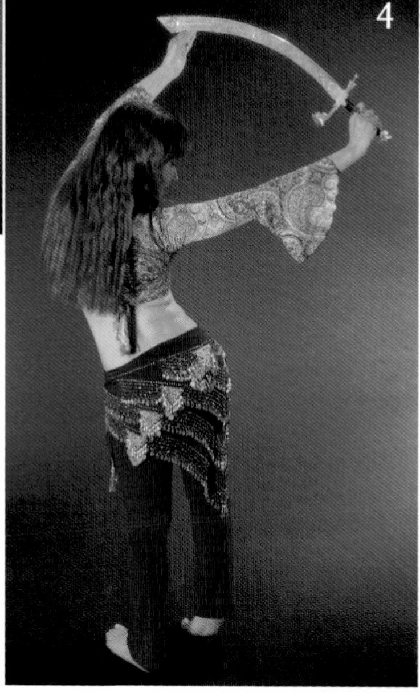

4 With small, delicate steps, slowly begin a spin. It is important to use the raising and lowering of your feet during the hip rolls to your advantage by working your steps in time with the rise and fall. When your foot pulls up for the hip roll, just as it reaches the top of the ball, lift it a small amount and take a step in the direction you want to spin. Lower the full foot to the ground. As you lift your other foot for the hip circle to the other side, repeat the step, again lowering the full foot to the ground afterwards. Continue this stepping in the direction you want to spin and you will find yourself in a full triple circle: one with your hips, one with your sword and one with your body.

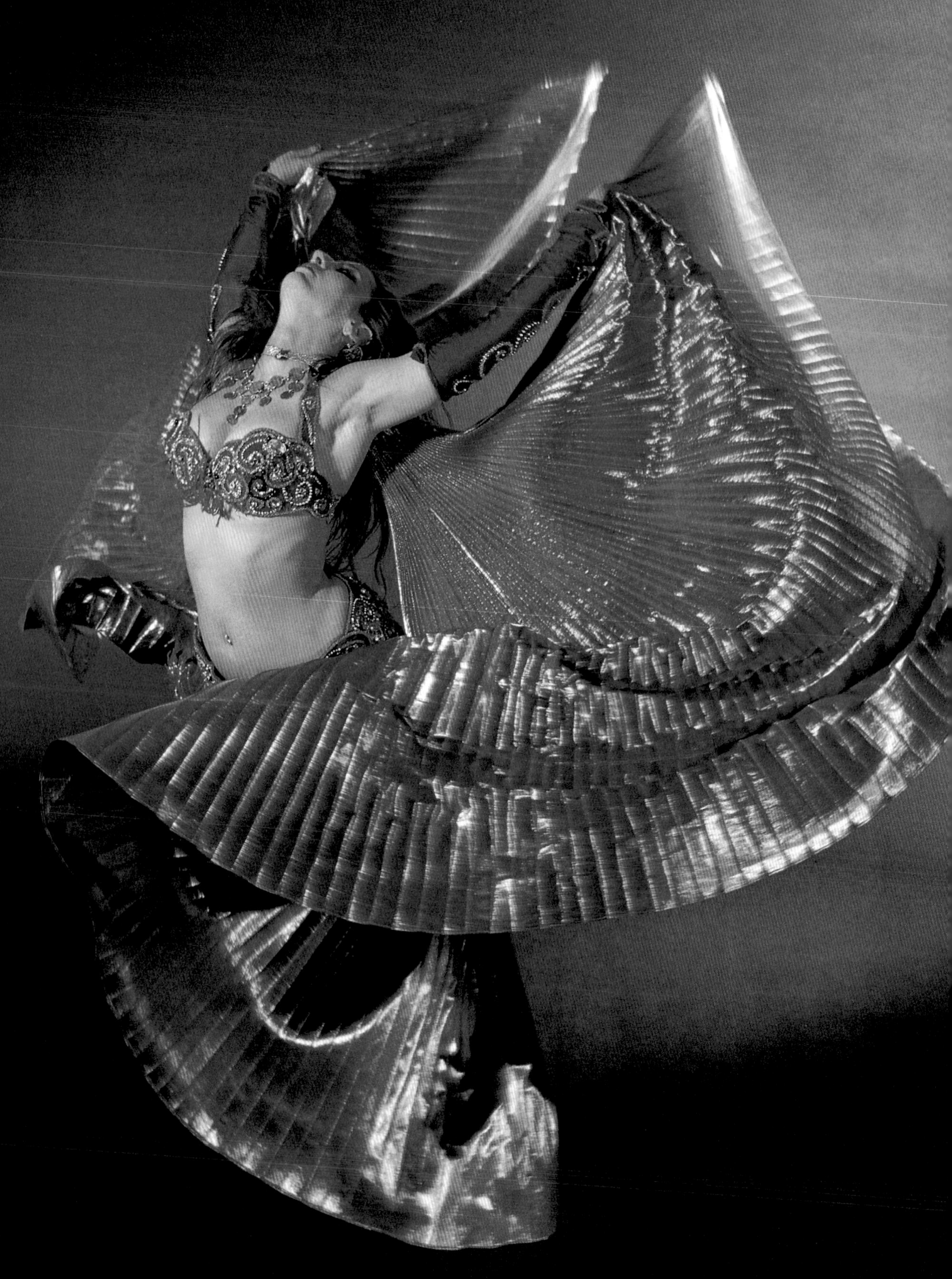

6 Wings

Drama, beauty and an incredible delight for the eyes are just a few of the words that spring to mind when describing wings. To dance with wings is to feel like a queen before all of humanity, a rose amid brambles, or streaming silk on rough burlap. Although wings are a modern addition to the world of belly dance, they manage to conjure up images of the great pharaohs, terrible gods and temperamental goddesses of Ancient Egypt.

There are two types of wings currently used by belly dancers. The style you choose will depend to some extent on the concept you'd like to convey. In one type, the wings wrap around the upper arm over the bicep and tricep muscles and conjure a look reminiscent of the glorious hieroglyphs of herons and bird deities on the walls of the great temple of Karnak. The second type attaches around the neck like a gilded collar. The material left flowing behind looks like the monarch's cape displayed in so many etchings of the wealthy in Ancient Egypt.

Traditionally, wings were made of thick, but lightweight, gold or silver lamé. Now they are also available in a dazzling rainbow of colours, textures and fibres, ranging from the boldest of satins to subtle pastel chiffons. Each wing is constructed from a large semicircle of material with a complex pleated design pressed into it. The pleats allow for very small creases where the band attaches to the body and gradually grow larger toward the edges of the material. A long pocket is sewn into the upper edge of the wing for a wooden dowel to be inserted. The dowel not only allows you to grasp the wing and keep it stable but also acts as an extension of your arm, creating extraordinary reach. When the wings are extended, the length and symmetrical folds of the fabric create an illusion of feathers catching the wind while in movement.

The dramatic scale and appearance of wings makes them a wonderful accompaniment to your dancing but also restricts their use. It's almost impossible to practice wing techniques at home because you need somewhere with a high ceiling and a great deal of empty space. Most dancers rent studio space for wing practice. Actual performances with wings are rare because only a full stage or a large restaurant with plenty of space can accommodate them.

Regardless of these obstacles, wings are an integral component of your dance practice so do your best to learn them. Whichever design or material you choose, wherever you find to dance, one of the most delightful aspects about dancing with wings is that almost everything you manage to do with them is shatteringly gorgeous – an eye-popping, jaw-dropping, heart-pounding spectacle!

GETTING FAMILIAR WITH WINGS

The best way to begin learning wings is just to play with them. Imagine you are a little girl again and someone has given you a pair of wings. You would probably run round the house trying to fly. Well, do just that now – play with your wings, swing them, circle them, flap them. Let your imagination soar for a few minutes as you experiment. This activity will help you grow accustomed to the feel and dynamics of dancing with wings.

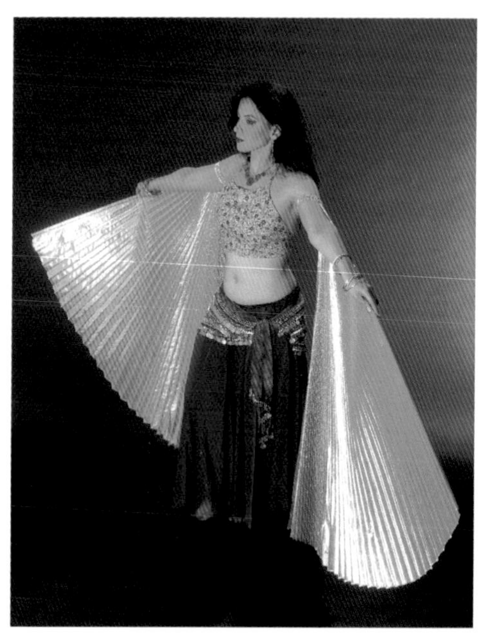

HOW TO HOLD WINGS

Stand in the basic foundation pose (p.20), but with your arms at your sides. With the wings hanging loose, manoeuvre the fabric until it is behind the dowels. With the dowels in the front of the wings, grab each one firmly, with knuckles facing out. You are ready to begin total wing enchantment!

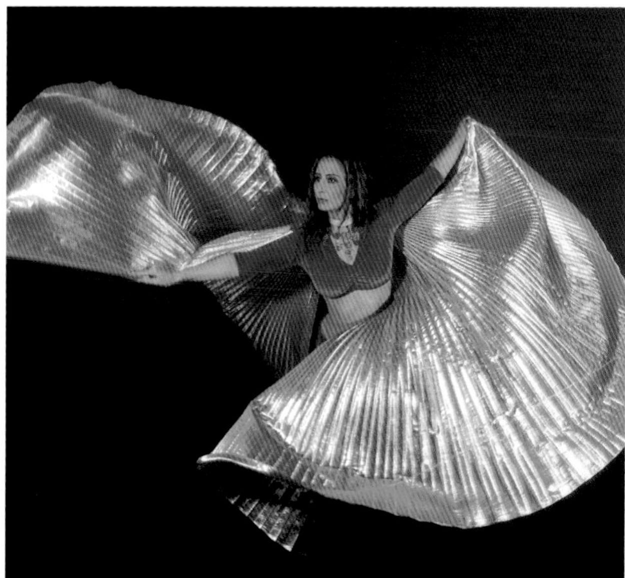

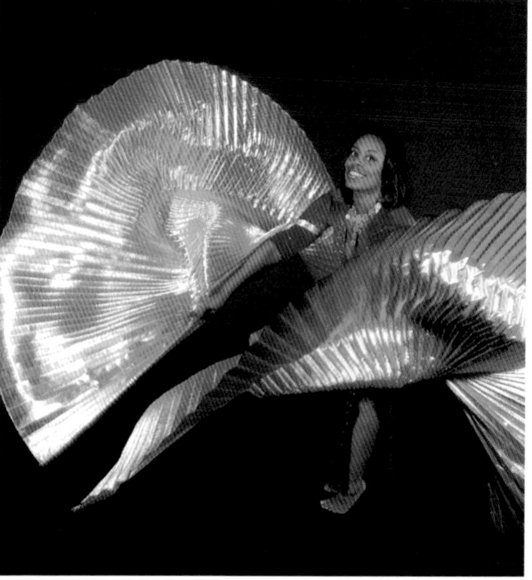

EXPERIMENTATION

Turn in circles, watching your wings billow out. Swing your arms back and forth, marvelling at the dancing fabric. By experimenting, you can develop fun movements and poses that are all your own. But do write down any interesting steps you discover before you forget them.

POSES

The wings are so spectacular that simple poses can be a primary part of any wing piece. Adding poses in between steps is a perfect way to accent the exciting, flowing beauty of the wings.

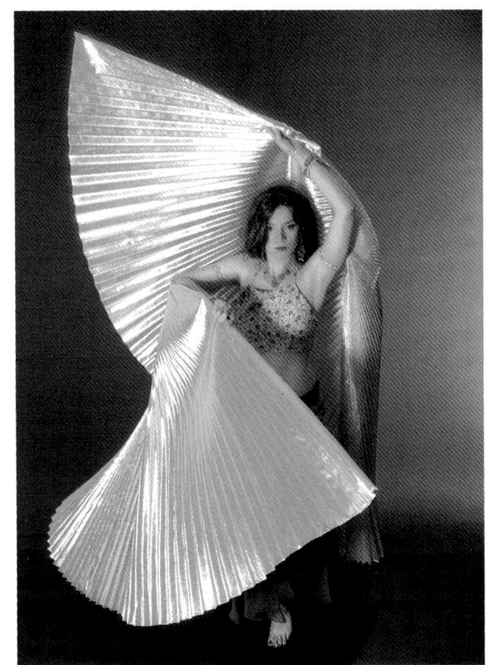

THE HATHOR

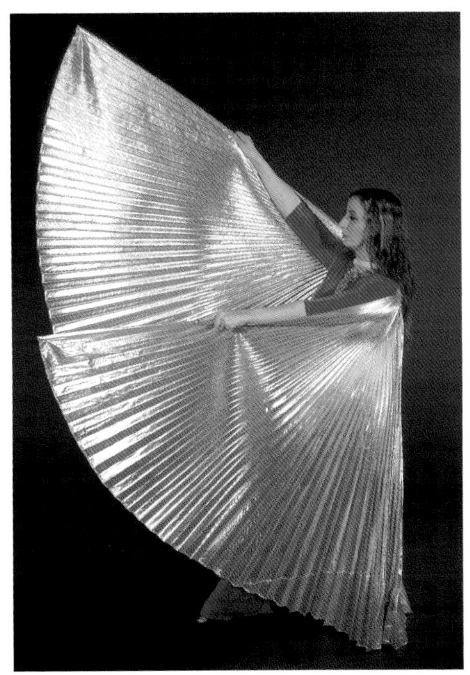

THE ISIS

THE OSIRIS

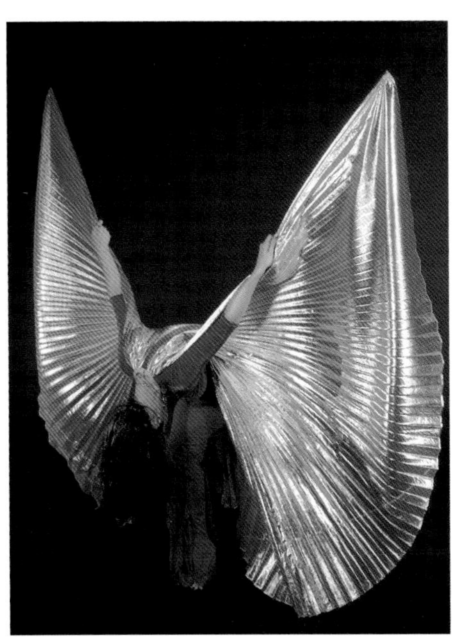

THE HORUS

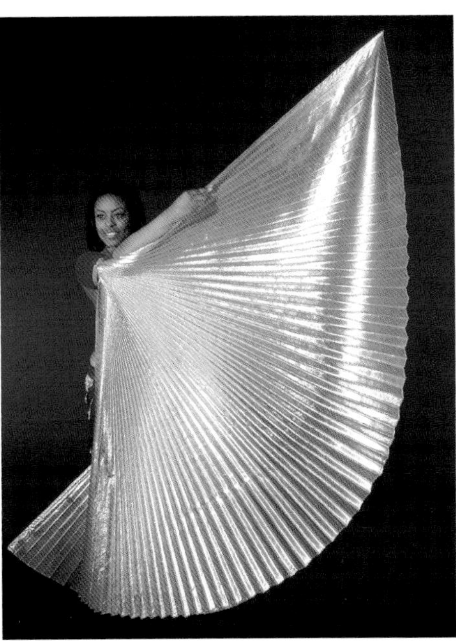

HALO TURN

1 Begin by spinning slowly, using small steps, around to the left. As your body begins to turn, drop your left arm in a circular sweep downward and raise your right arm in a circular sweep upward. Continue to sweep your arms around until you are facing the back of your dance space and both your arms are up in the air circling toward the right.

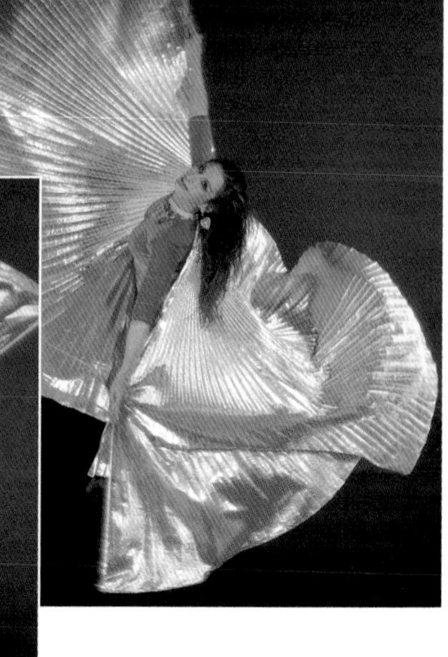

2 As you spin forward, begin sweeping your right arm in an arc downward, crossing in front of your body, followed by your left. Keep spinning your body and circling your arms while gaining in speed. The wings will whip round you, creating an amazing full body halo.

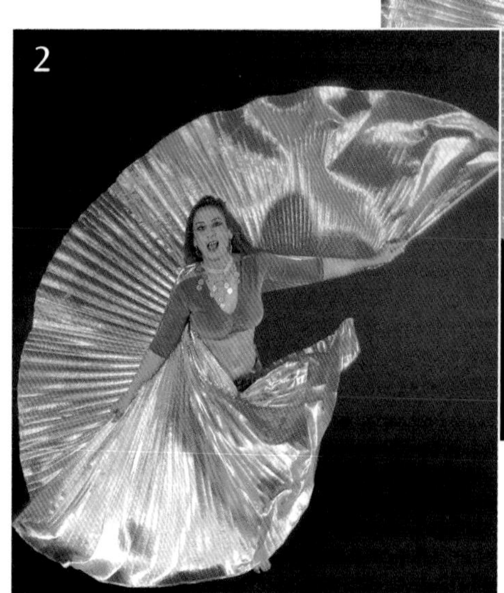

COCOON

1 Raise your arms up and out at your sides, keeping your elbows locked. Stop when your arms are parallel to the floor. Keeping your wrists perfectly straight, bend your elbows until the wings are very close to your body, like a cocoon.

2 Begin spinning with small steps. The wings will catch the air and the flowing material will cover you demurely, front and back, while allowing the briefest glimpses of your face. To finish with a flourish, bring both arms down to each side with energy and speed. Then sweep the wings forward, out to the side and up, holding them high for drama!

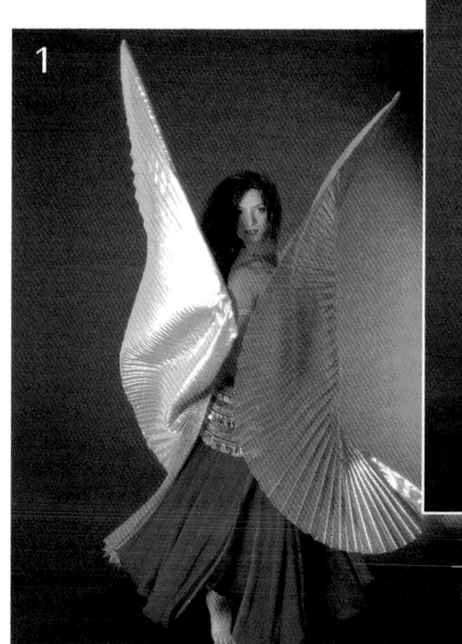

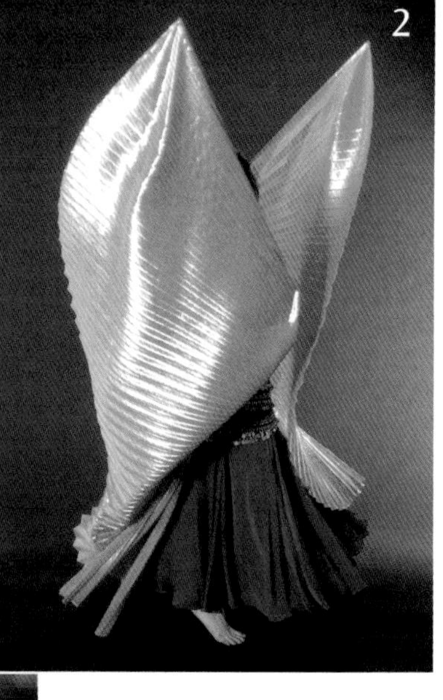

WING SWISH

1 Grasping the dowels from the outside, raise your right arm high, extending it diagonally from the shoulder. Cross your left arm delicately across your lower body.

2 Quickly wave your right arm in a wide semi-circular movement down and across your body to the left.

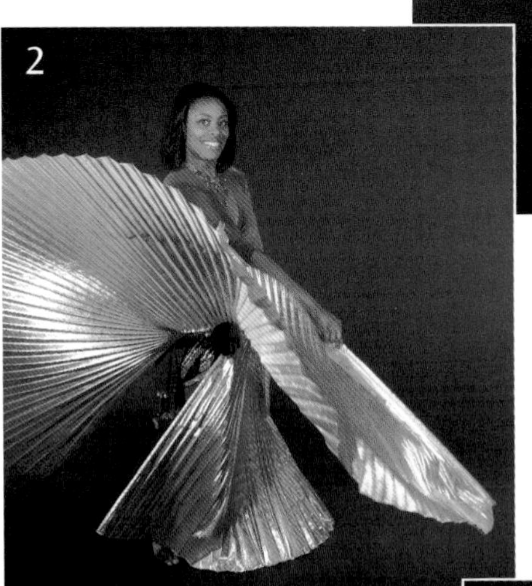

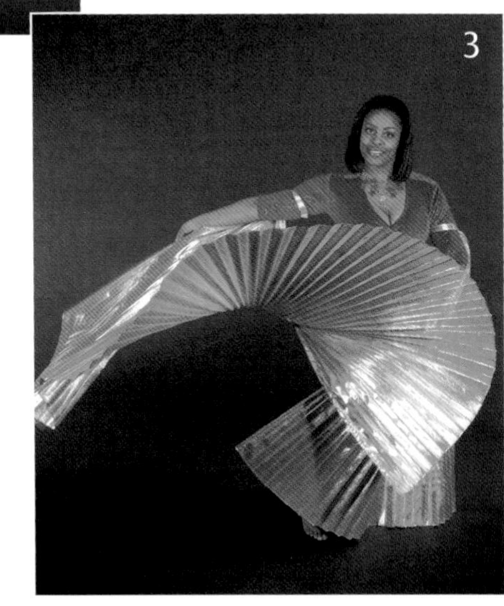

3 When your right wing has gone as low and as far left as your arm can take, twist your wrist until your palm turns over and wave the wing up and back to the right. The entire step will take two counts: one count for the swish forward and one for the swish back. When done continuously, the wing should look as if it is forming a figure eight horizontally with the floor. Repeat the movement with your left wing.

PRACTICE

Swish the wings one at a time, starting on the right for four full steps. Then switch to the left and swish four times. Then bring both arms together and perform two full simultaneous swishes.

THE PROUD/MOURNFUL HERON

1 Start in a right leg foundation (p.20). Hold the wings up high on each side of your body. With your left foot, take a large step, 1.2m (4ft) or so, forward. Keep your spine straight and stretch your arms out and behind you.

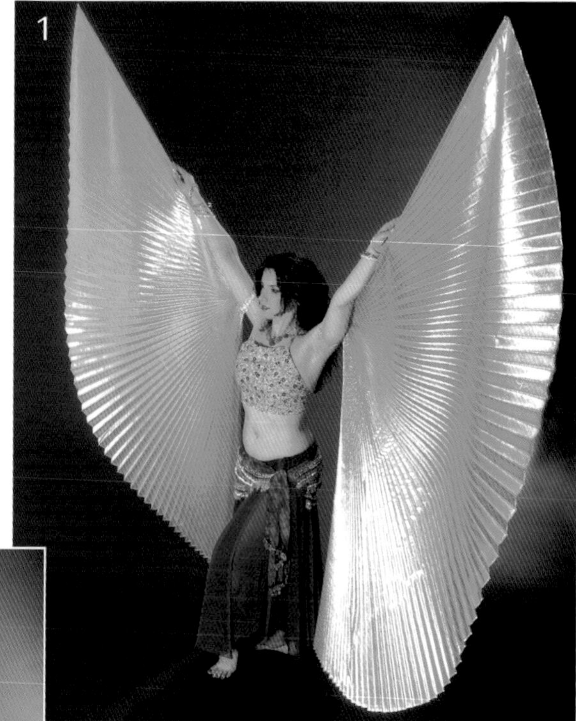

2 Simultaneously bend your left knee as much as you can, keeping your right leg almost straight, until you are very close to the ground in a deep forward lunge. Keeping your arms straight, curl your body forward while swinging the wings gently up, then forward and down in a large beautiful arc.

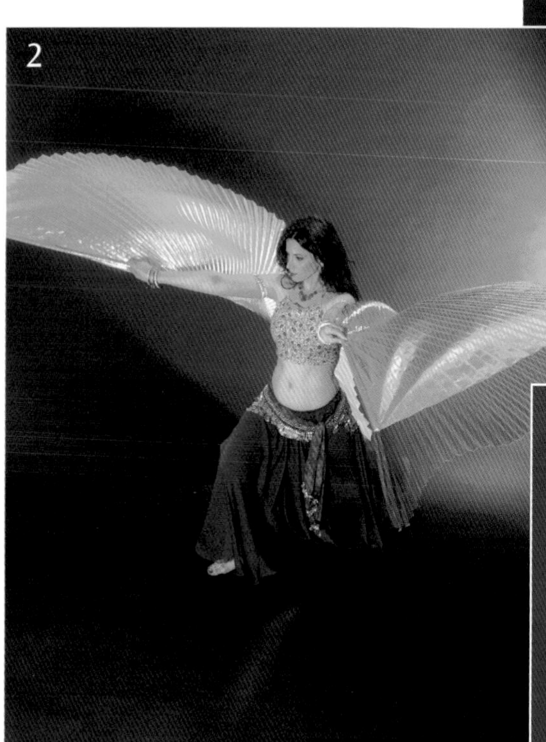

3 As the wings descend, curve your body forward as far as you can, dipping your head down to face the ground and rolling your shoulders in. The very tips of the wings should almost touch the floor.

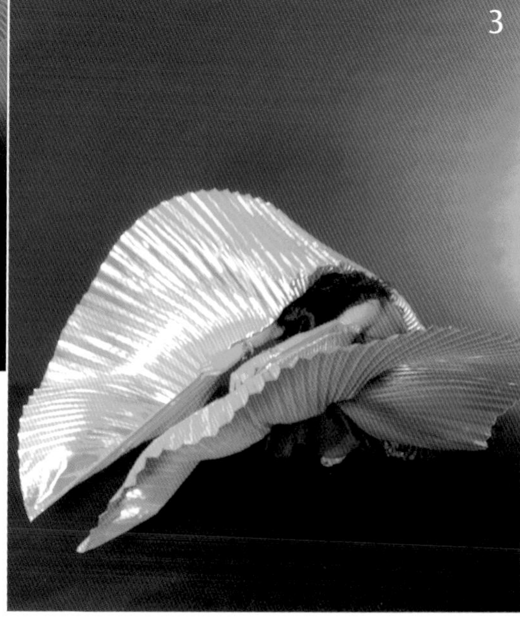

TIP

If your legs are not very strong, you should only lunge a little until your body builds the strength it needs to sink all the way down. If you have any back pain, injury or weakness, don't do the backbend.

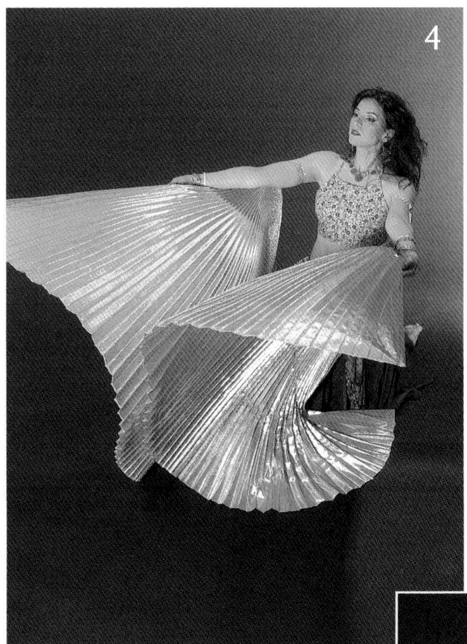

4 Suddenly straighten your back and, at the same time, swing the wings up to shoulder level. Crest the wings outward at a gentle descending angle.

5 Keeping the fluidity of the movement, tilt your head and body backward and finally sweep the wings into a high wide arc behind you. Step back and repeat on the right side, starting with your right foot.

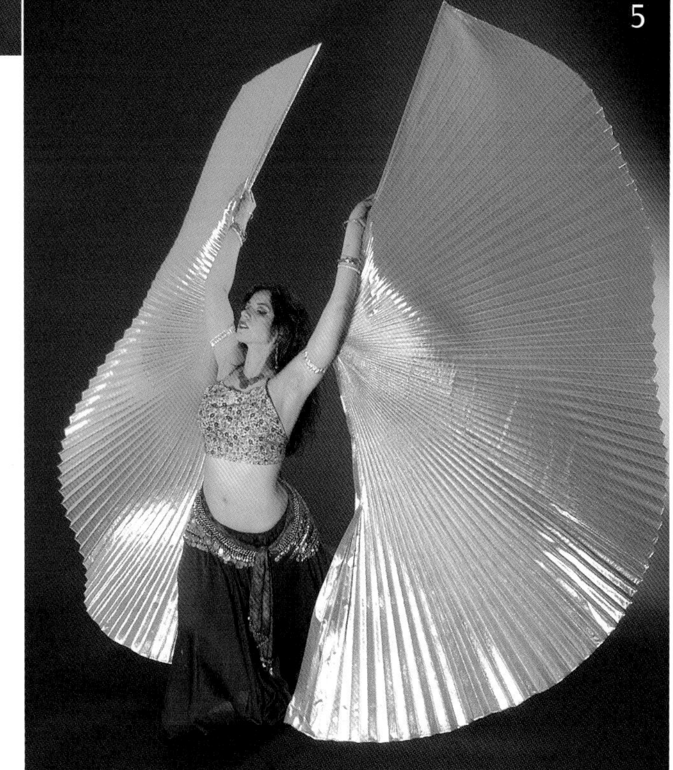

ADDING EMOTION

This versatile wing step can be used in both playful and solemn dances. All the dancer has to do is to make some small alterations in her expression to change the feeling of the dance.

To make this step playful, hop into the lunge and quickly rise up from the forward sweep with a jolt of energy, happy eyes and a wide joyful grin.

To create a mournful mood, dance the entire step with thoughtful deliberation. Relax your face muscles so there isn't the slightest hint of tension. While sliding into the lunge, peer down so that you are looking at the floor until the wings begin to come up and back. When the wings are just about at the final proud heron stage, throw your head back and switch your gaze from the ground to the ceiling. Repeat this in the other direction.

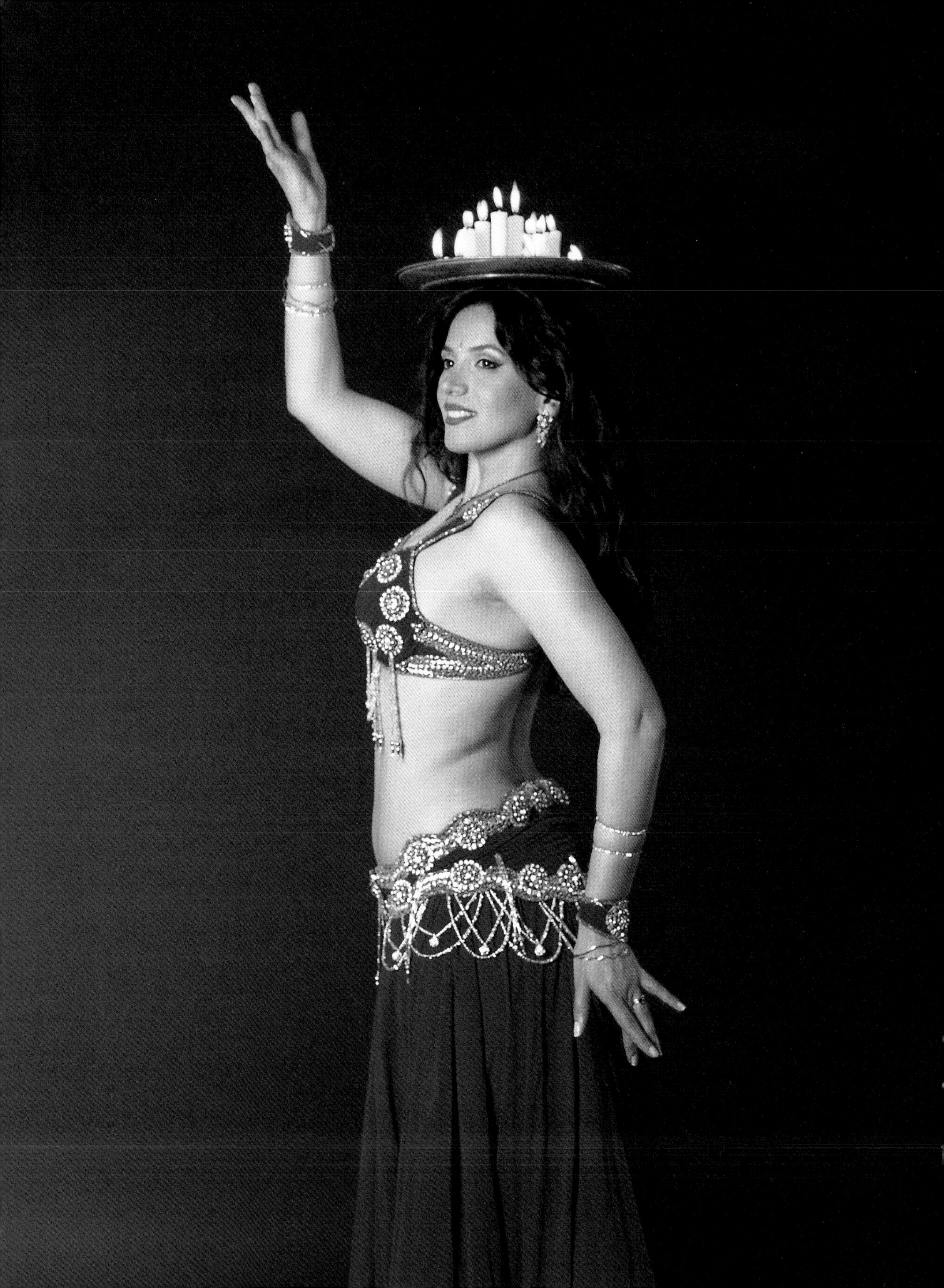

7 Variety: the spice of life

As well as the sword, veil and wings, there are a number of other props you can use to create interest and drama in your dance.

CANDLES

These are very popular props. Most candle dancers work with a large silver tray, bearing candles in all shapes and sizes, which they balance on their head. Dancing with a tray of fire on your head is at once terrifying and awesome – a technique certainly worth learning! As with the sword, candles can be dangerous if not handled correctly, so take care. And for safety's sake, I recommend that you keep a fire extinguisher in your dance space with you, especially while learning. Take your time when selecting your tray and if you want to start out with something fancy, go ahead. It needn't be brand new. In fact, some of the most beautiful and charming trays I have seen have been old, bought at second-hand shops or antique markets.

CANE

Dancing with a cane may have its roots in a masculine battle dance, or *tahtiyb,* from the Upper Egypt farmland regions. In a simulated fighting style, the men danced with long hardwood sticks, using powerful, aggressive movements. The mock skirmish consisted of much waving and striking of the sticks as well as energetic hops and leaps. Over time, a feminine adaptation emerged with a more lighthearted and playful style, substituting a delicate hooked cane for the stick. When choosing a cane, look for one that is long enough to lean on, narrow enough for your hand to grasp, and light enough for you to lift without effort.

FINGER CYMBALS

I like the Turkish name for these – *zills* – but they are known as *sil sil* in Arabic, *salasih* in Farsi and *zagat* in Egyptian. Musical instruments for fingers date back to 200 BC, when dancers in celebrations would clack together two wooden or ivory sticks in each hand. As cultures progressed, so did the quality of instrumentation. Some evidence suggests that it was the Greeks who first began playing a metal form of finger instrument, but nobody is sure. The only firm fact about finger cymbals is that learning to play them is HARD, but worth every ounce of effort.

Zills are a musical instrument, so it's important to select them for their sound, not beauty. Listen to them chime a few times before you buy and check they make a clear bell-like ring (not a clack) that resonates for at least three seconds after the strike. Generally the longer the sound resonates, the better the zills.

CANDLES

Dancing with a tray of candles requires the same care and concentration as dancing with a sword, and sword techniques (pp.98–107) can be used with candles. However, unlike the sword, you must hold the tray of candles firmly with both hands at all times – never with just fingers or one hand – to be sure you don't drop it and get burned.

As a beginner, don't light the candles until you are absolutely in control of the tray and feel no fear or insecurity about your skills. As for sword, the rule of thumb is when you can get through the entire candle lesson four times back to back without losing the tray even once, you can consider taking the leap to lighting the candles. When you do light them, don't immediately launch into a full routine. The fire on your head may make you nervous at first, so practice the movements, one at a time, very slowly until you feel comfortable. As your confidence grows, you can begin to put movements together to build a routine.

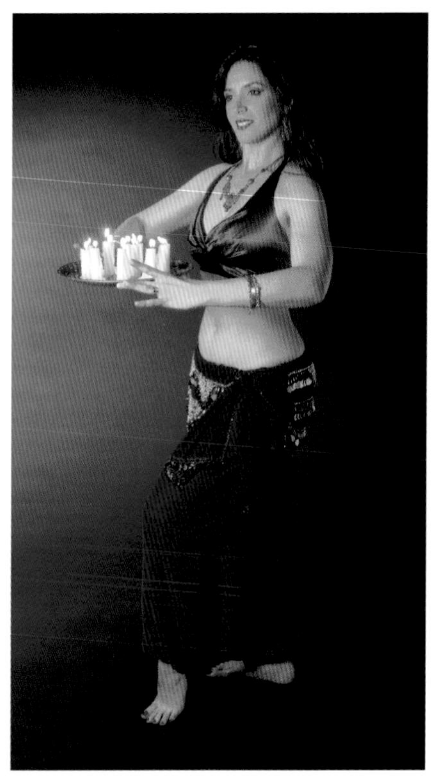

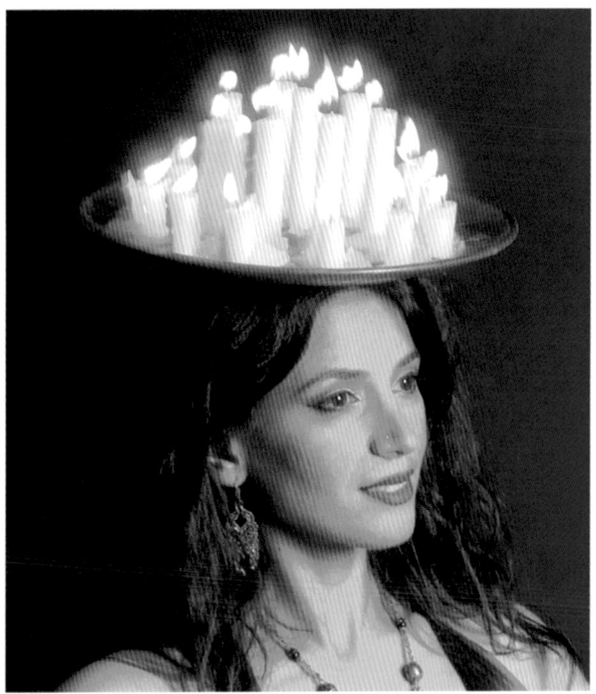

PLACING THE CANDLES

In order to balance the tray, it is vital to position the candles evenly. When choosing candles there are two options. You might like to choose one candle that has a large base measuring 5–7cm (2–3in) and is 10–15cm (4–6in) tall, with 15 or so more slender pillar candles of varying heights to place around it. Or you may prefer to use 20 pillars of different heights, carefully placed with the highest in the center and the shortest around the edges of the tray as shown here.

Fix the candles to the tray with candle adhesive or sticky tack. Do NOT light the candles.

NEONIC DROPS

This advanced step is named after the first dancer I ever saw perform it, while balancing a tray of 30 candles on her head. When she danced this step, the drop was so sudden and unexpected that it almost seemed as if she had tripped. The audience literally gasped in admiration. Such a step requires great skill and lots of practice but is well worth working for.

1 From foundation (p.20), step forward with your left foot, transferring 70 percent of your weight onto it. Without bouncing up first (as many people do) and knocking the tray off balance, immediately drop into deep lunge.

2 Slowly come back up in a reverse, well-controlled undulation. Beginning at the hips, curve in your waist and stomach.

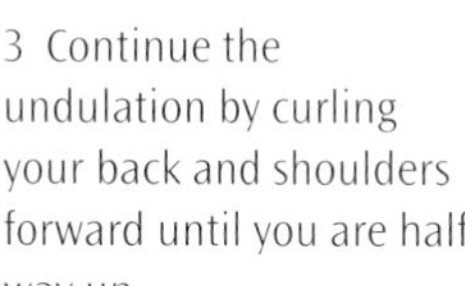

3 Continue the undulation by curling your back and shoulders forward until you are half way up.

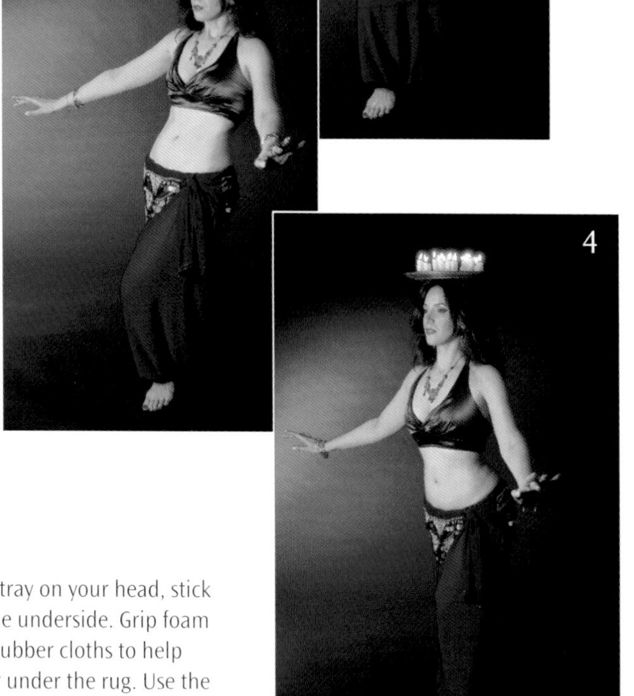

4 When the reverse undulation reaches your shoulders, first curl them in and then push forward, leading with your chest, while straightening your legs the rest of the way.

TIP

If you have trouble keeping a tray on your head, stick a thin piece of grip foam to the underside. Grip foam is the material used to make rubber cloths to help open jars or non-skid pads for under the rug. Use the smallest amount possible to secure the tray to your head so it is as inconspicuous as possible.

PRACTICE

Step forward with your right foot and repeat the drop and reverse undulation. Practice this step around your dance space.

KNEE WALK

Whenever I see this step, I always think of youthful temple daughters worshipping their goddess during a ritual by bowing down on their knees in respect and adoration. In more practical terms, the knee walk is a great way to take you across the floor without interrupting a floor routine.

TIP
While learning this step, wear knee pads to avoid bruising or injury. When practicing or performing the knee walk, wear harem pants in slippery fabric or some other leg covering. The fabric will protect your skin from chafing and burns from the floor when you slide.

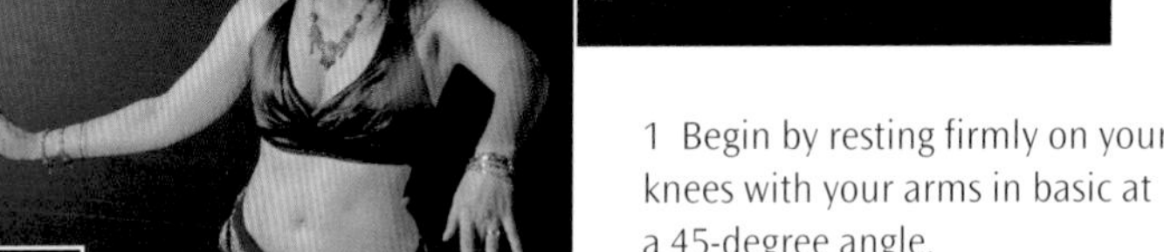

1 Begin by resting firmly on your knees with your arms in basic at a 45-degree angle.

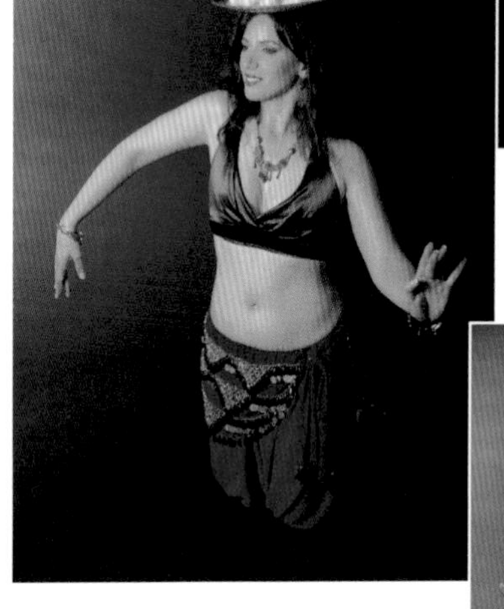

2 Slide your left knee forward and diagonally to the left, forcing your body into a deep lunge. Simultaneously begin a left snake arm (p.54), reaching out in the same direction as your knee.

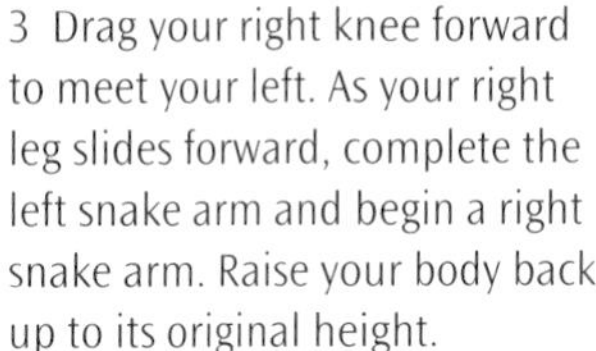

3 Drag your right knee forward to meet your left. As your right leg slides forward, complete the left snake arm and begin a right snake arm. Raise your body back up to its original height.

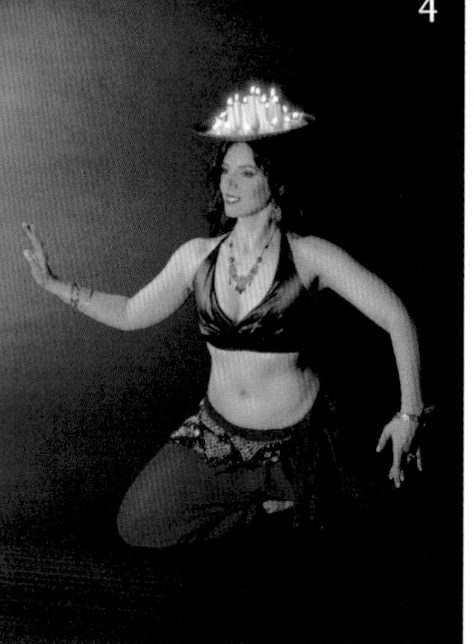

4 Slide your right knee forward and diagonally to the right. This will once again force your body into a deep lunge. Complete the right snake arm and begin another on the left as you drag your left knee to the right, returning to the starting position.

BACKBEND UNDULATION

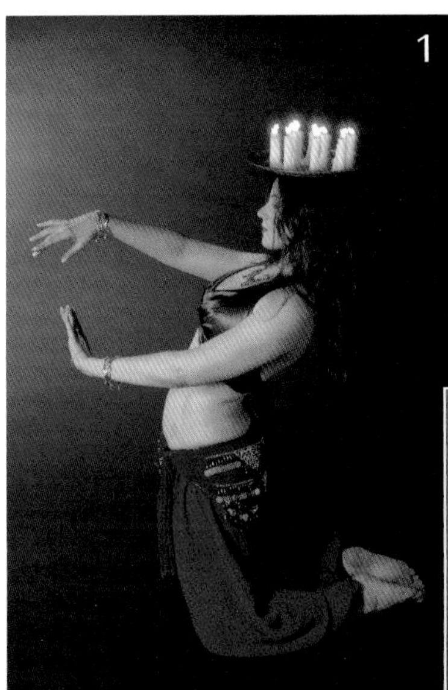

1 Start in the same position as for the knee walk, but turn your body to profile. Spread your knees apart a full 1.2m (4ft) while touching your toes together behind you. This triangular leg support spreads your body weight to help maintain balance. Begin snaking both arms forward.

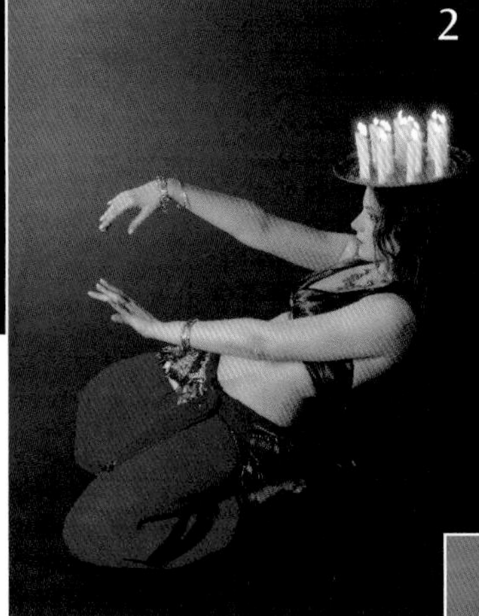

2 Keeping your chin parallel with the floor, lean back as far as you can without strain, supporting yourself with your thigh muscles. Keep snaking your arms in front of you – they are a convenient counterbalance to the force of gravity pulling you backward.

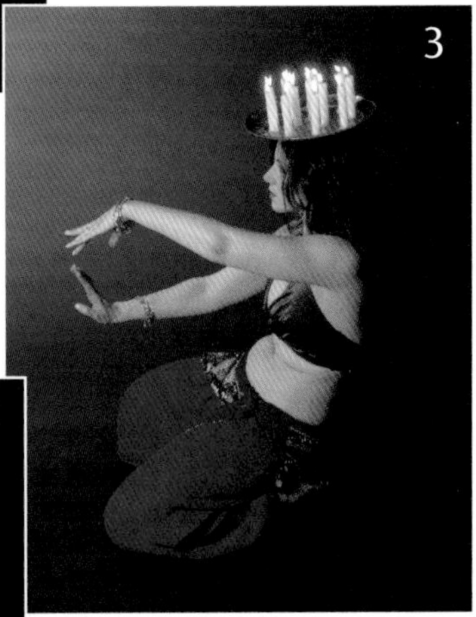

3. Hunch your shoulders slightly and curl your upper body forward – don't just pop straight up – pulling in your abdominal muscles while almost sitting fully on your feet.

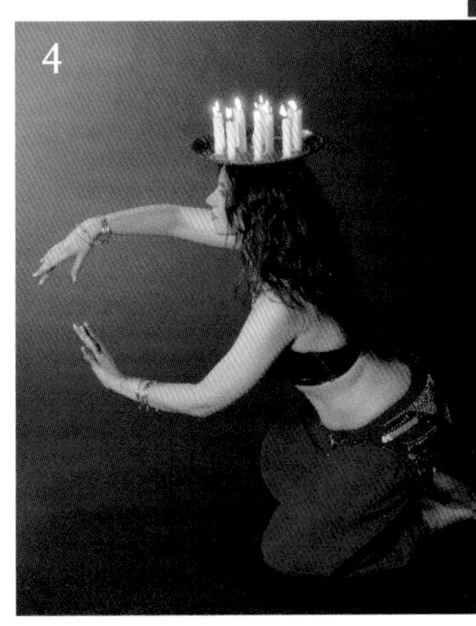

4 When your upper body is directly over your knees, lift up off your feet, roll your shoulders back and push your chest forward. Arch your back and come up from the sitting position by leading forward and upward with your chest. Return to the starting position and repeat!

WARNING
As with all backbends, perform this movement slowly and with extreme care to avoid injuring your back.

CANE STEPS

LEAPING SKIP STEP

1 Hold the base of the cane with your right hand and the crook with your left. Stand in right foot foundation with the cane at chest level in front of you. Turn slightly to the left until the right side of your body is somewhat forward. With a small hop, jump forward and as you land, bend your knees to lower your body into a dip. Try not to lean forward as you dip, just lower your center of gravity. Lift the cane up above your head.

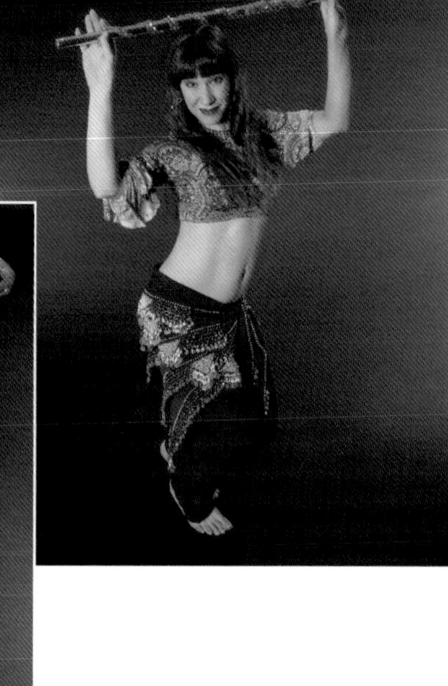

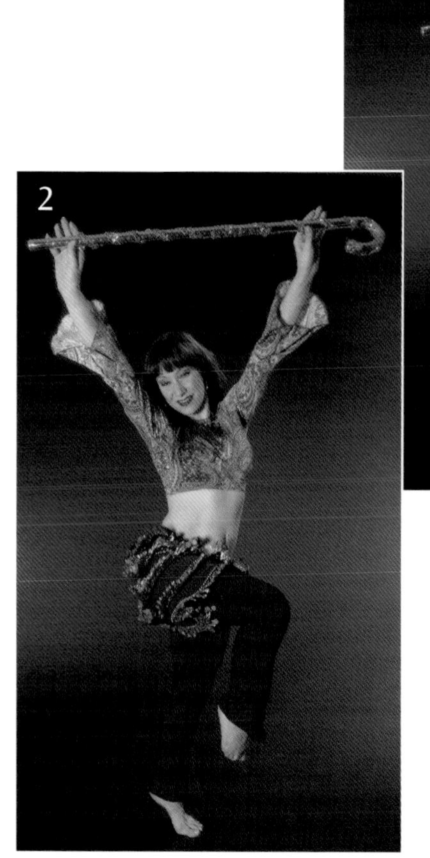

2 Follow the dip with a fast energetic leap straight up into a left foot releve (p.56). At the same time, bend your right knee, raise your leg with a hip lift and straighten your arms to hold the cane high above your head.

As you descend, lower your arms back to chest level and pivot to the right until the left side of your body is slightly facing front. Repeat the movement on the other side.

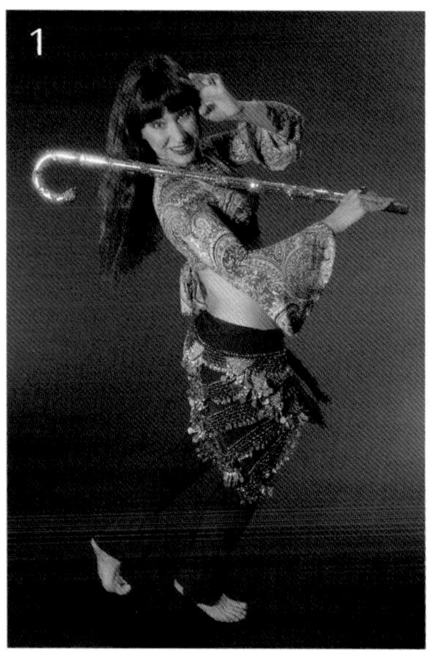

HIP PUSH STEP

1 Start in the same position as for the leaping skip step, but hold only the bottom of the cane in your right hand. Rest the crook on your right shoulder.

Softly extend the first finger of your left hand while curling over the others. Rest the side of your forefinger against the left side of your forehead in a delicate salute.

2 Lifting your right leg and bending at the knee, hip snap (p.30) to the back. On the release of the snap, place your right foot forward, about 30cm (12in) past your left, and hip snap forward on your right side. Repeat four times, then switch to the other side for another four.

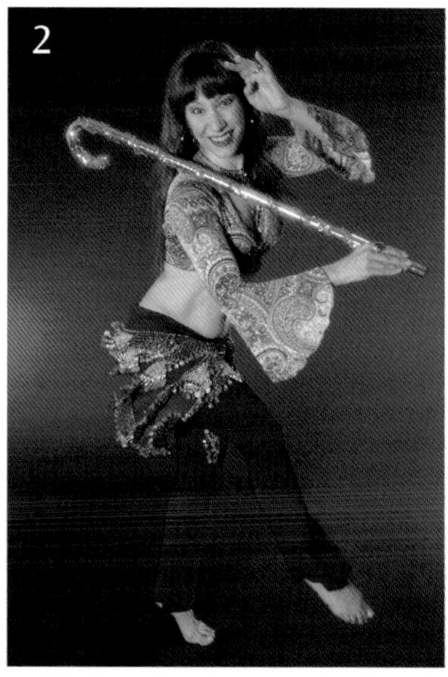

SWINGING THE CANE: PREPARATION

Grasp the cane firmly, 5cm (2in) from the bottom, with your dominant hand. Your fingers should be firmly wrapped round the entire stalk. Swing the cane round twice in a clockwise direction, without relaxing your grip. Reverse and swing counterclockwise. Notice that your wrist has trouble spinning gracefully with the cane and torques uncomfortably left and right. The following steps demonstrate how to twirl a cane smoothly without strain on your wrist.

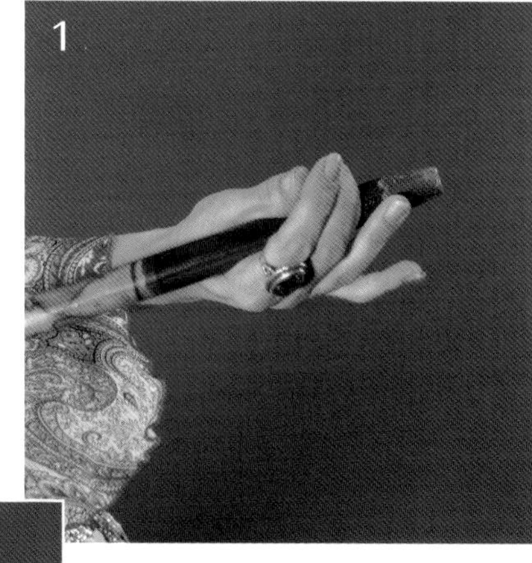

SWINGING THE CANE

1 Grasp the cane firmly. Release all fingers except your forefinger and thumb and keep a firm grip with those.

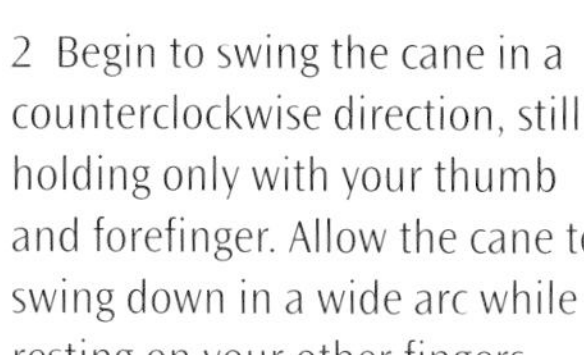

2 Begin to swing the cane in a counterclockwise direction, still holding only with your thumb and forefinger. Allow the cane to swing down in a wide arc while resting on your other fingers.

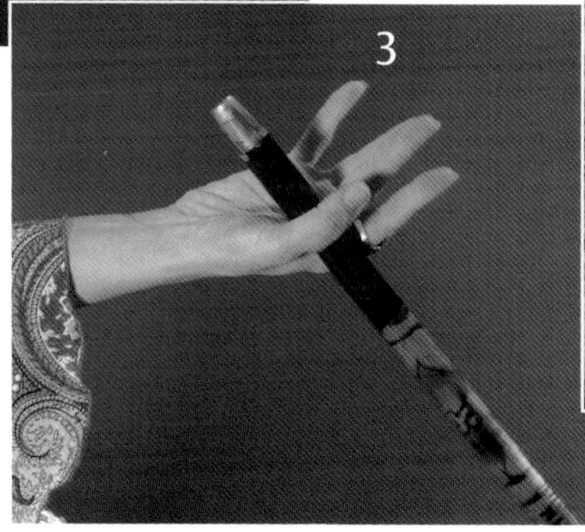

3 As the cane begins to swing up, the end will lift off the fingers it's resting on. Extend those fingers, preparing for the final step.

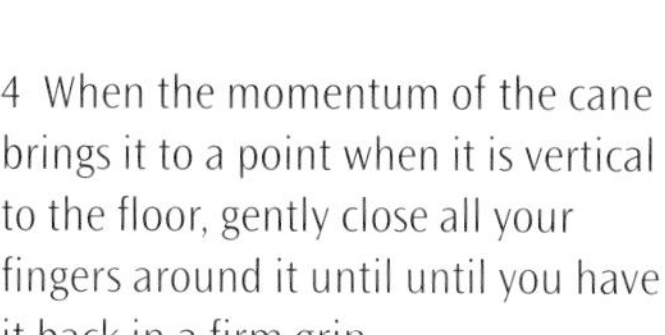

4 When the momentum of the cane brings it to a point when it is vertical to the floor, gently close all your fingers around it until until you have it back in a firm grip.

PRACTICE

Spin the cane slowly and carefully, making one spin at a time and pausing before the next, until you feel comfortable. Then start spinning the cane more rapidly, removing the pauses so that one spin flows seamlessly into the next. For a final experiment, spin the cane once on your right side. Then, keeping it in the same hand, cross your arm over your chest to the opposite side and swing the cane once on the left side. Repeat.

ZILLS

Often viewed as just another prop to the dance, many dancers forget that zills, or finger cymbals, are a musical instrument and require practice to master. Poorly played zills can, and will, undermine even the greatest of dancers. But I urge you to not be afraid! Embrace the zills, practice and the payback will be tremendous.

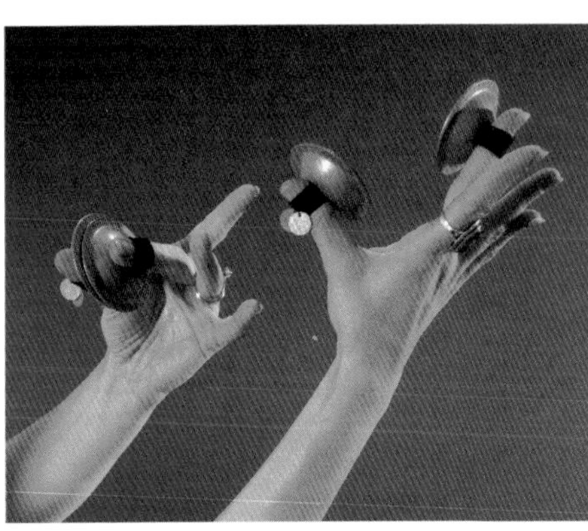

WEARING THE ZILLS

You need two sets of zills for proper instrumentation. A zill should be attached to your thumb and middle finger by elastic running through the hole at the top of the zill. One technique is to run a loop of elastic through the hole, measure it to your finger and tie a knot on the inside of the zill. Another is to use small safety pins to hold the elastic in place. The zills should fit tightly but not be so tight that the tips of your fingers turn blue. If necessary, loosen the elastic. Like different notes, zill chimes vary in strength and style.

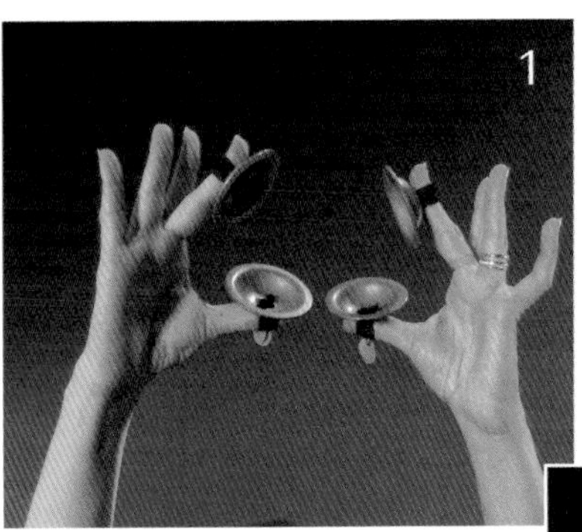

BASIC RING

1 Position the zills on the thumb and middle finger of each hand.

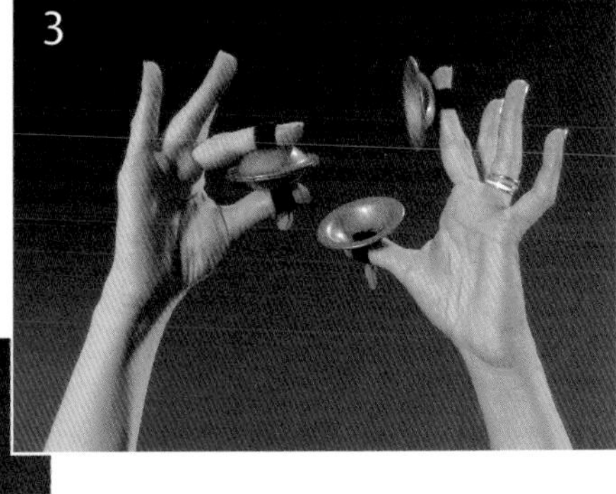

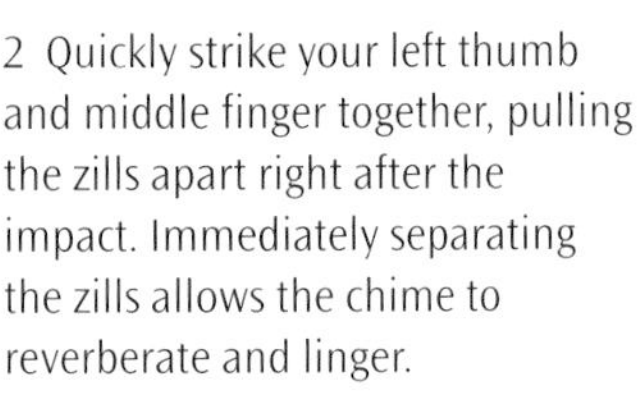

2 Quickly strike your left thumb and middle finger together, pulling the zills apart right after the impact. Immediately separating the zills allows the chime to reverberate and linger.

3 Repeat with your right hand.

PRACTICE

Ring the zills in each hand slowly, one after another, allowing the chime to linger. Speed up gradually, striking left then right until you have a steady rapid pace. Stop. Begin again, but ring the zills softly at first, building in volume by adding pressure to each strike.

WIND CHIME

Hold your zills apart in each hand, palm up, with your left hand in front of your right. Move your left hand directly toward you, and your right hand directly away from you so that the edges of the left zills strike the edges of the right zills as they pass each other, moving in opposite directions. This will create a magical wind-chiming effect, which seems almost fairylike. Repeat the set to practice and perfect your technique.

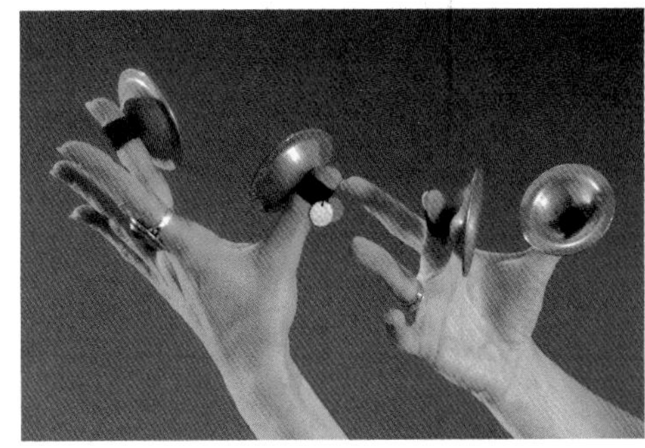

SAMPLE RHYTHMS

Practice to a slow drumbeat from your favourite music.
For 8 drumbeats, single strike your right zill only once on each beat. Repeat on the left.
For the next 8 beats, quickly double strike (R,L) on each beat.
Finally, for another 8 beats, quickly triple strike (R,L,R) on each beat.

Traditional gallop 8 counts, one set of strikes per drumbeat:
Triple strike, triple strike, triple strike… (RLR, RLR, RLR).

Rolling gallop 13 very fast alternating single strikes for every 8 counts:
Single strike R, single strike L, single strike R… (R,L,R,L,R,L,R,L,R,L,R,L,R).

Beladi 9/8 count beat using single and triple strikes:
This is a tough one to teach in a book, so forgive this silly technique, but it works!
Strike R, Strike R, Holy Cow (R,L,R), Strike R, Holy Cow (R,L,R), Strike R, Strike L.
In other words: (R, L, R-L-R, R, R-L-R, R,L).

Chiftitelli 8-count accent rhythm with pauses:
Triple strike, triple strike, triple strike, single, single, single
(R-L-R, R-L-R, R-L-R, pause, R, R, R). Or:
Single strike, double strike, double strike, pause, single, single single
(R, RL, RL, pause, R, R, R).

USING ZILLS IN THE DANCE

A dancer can't just play zills – she has to play them and dance to their music. Stand in place and begin to play a steady single strike beat. March on the spot to it. Increase to double and then triple strike beat while continuing to march. After 16 triple strikes, begin to march forward and around your dance space while triple striking. Not as easy as it sounds.

As you get better at marching to the triple beat, try different steps such as the ghawazee step (p.61) and hip twist (p.36). When you have successfully combined those steps with zill playing – this takes some time, so don't lose hope – move on to playing other rhythms with the zills.

Practice will make perfect. If you're really struggling, don't get frustrated and give up. Keep playing and it will all come together.

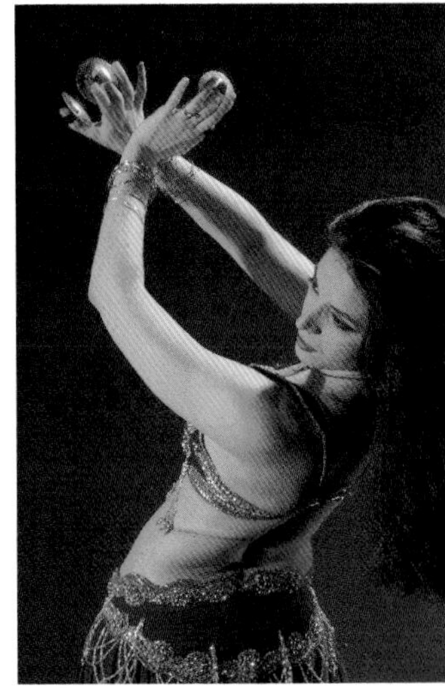

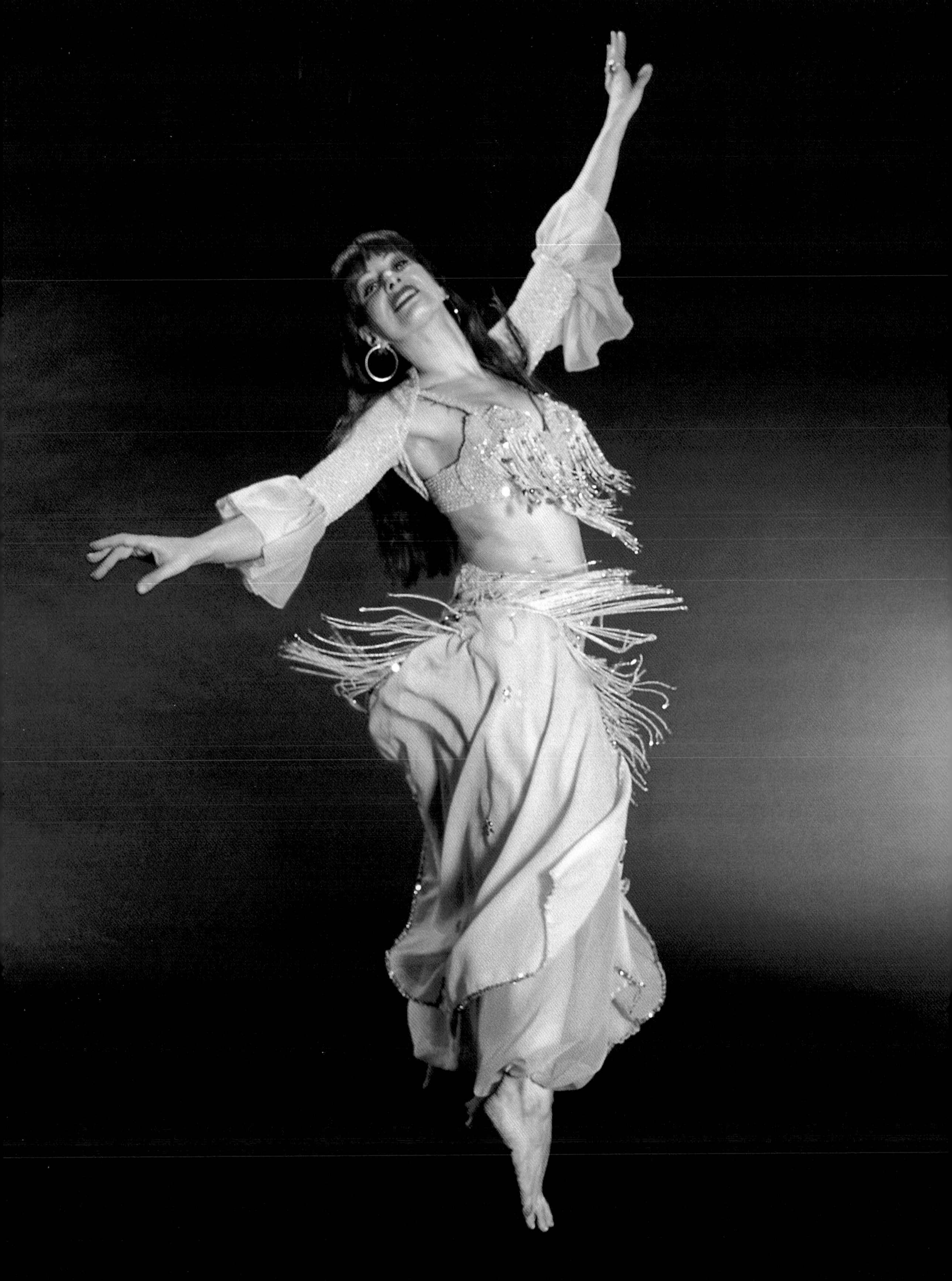

8 The Oriental fantasy

Thomas Alva Edison said, “Genius is one percent inspiration, 99 percent perspiration”. Belly dancing is no different. With the solid foundation of steps taught in the previous chapters, there is no limit to how much dancing you can do. The best way to improve your dancing is to practice, practice, practice! Each time you rehearse your dance steps, your body will grow more familiar with the movements and they will get easier and easier. One of the most enjoyable ways to practice, rather than just repeating each step over and over, is to build a dance routine. The routine brings all the steps together and blends them into one flowing dance.

Before I was a professional dancer, I spent many happy hours alone in my living room, dancing my heart out to the routines I developed. After a year or so, I began to feel a compelling desire to share my dancing with other people. Being an incurable romantic, I wanted to give them a chance to escape from their everyday lives into the magic of an Oriental dream. I wanted to take them with me to the places I went in my mind while I was dancing. Perhaps by now you might be feeling the same thing.

If you’re thinking about performing for other people, you’re probably feeling a strange mix of emotions – excitement, curiosity, suspense and hope, mingled with nervousness, insecurity and fear. Some people refer to the latter as stage fright. Revel in all the positive emotions and let them inspire you! As for the negative emotions, there are some really easy techniques to help you manage them.

OVERCOMING YOUR FEARS

Many beginners worry about what people will think when they see them dance for the first time. An easy remedy for stage fright is to invite only people you know and trust to your early performances. Family and close friends are excellent support for the fledgling dancer. If you’re planning to dance in a public place for the first time you might worry about what strangers will think about you and your dancing. Well, there are two types of people in the world as it relates to belly dancing – those who know how to belly dance and those who don’t. For those who don’t, anything you do is going to be marvellous because they don’t know any better. And those who do belly dance remember how it felt to be new and will be compassionate.

Another common phobia is the fear of forgetting the steps of the dance. There is only one cure for that – practice! If you keep rehearsing a routine, your body and mind will reach a point where the movements become second nature. The thought processes of which step comes after which will melt away as your body takes over and gets you moving.

BUILDING A ROUTINE

Many teachers propose different formulas for dancing which include some components and exclude others, based on their personal vision of belly dancing. It seems, however, that the most creative and talented dancers do not allow themselves to be limited by convention. They incorporate all their scope and talent, adding a touch of their own personality to the routine. With that in mind, I suggest a six-segment routine which touches on all your new skills as a dancer as a great place to begin.

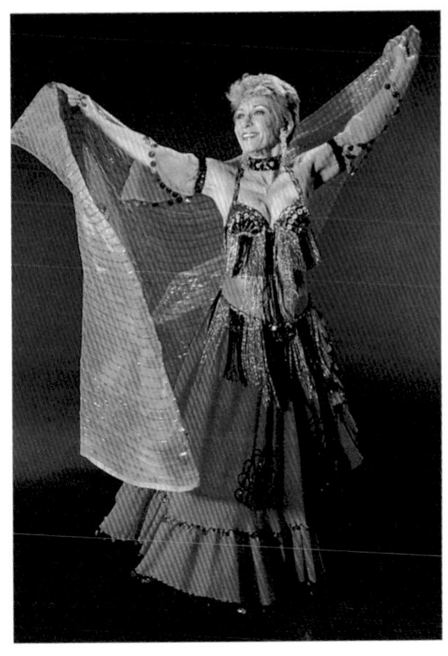

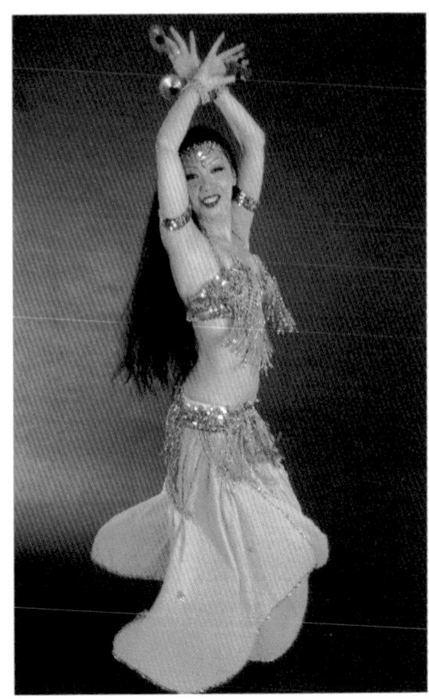

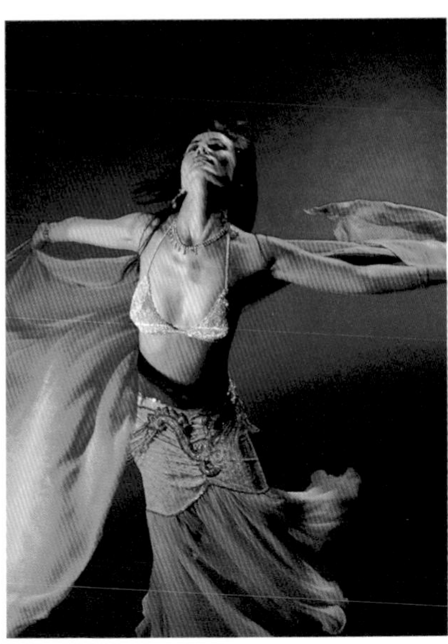

ENTRANCE (1–2 minutes)
The entrance, as you move into your dancing space, is as much a part of the dance as anything else. It's generally best to use graceful arm movements and dramatized walks and save everything else for the body of the routine. Enter slowly and moodily, using the pharonic walk (p.59), or leap into position with joy, using the ghawazee step (p.61).

DANCING OR ZILL SET (2–4 minutes)
As the entrance concludes, the first full dance piece is perfect for energetic dancing, with or without the chiming of zills to get you, and any audience, revved up. Zills add vigour and life to a speedy opening number.

VEIL (4–5 minutes)
Nobody likes to see the same dance over and over. Changing the mood by moving into veil work, light and ethereal as an evening summer breeze, will add some depth and variety.

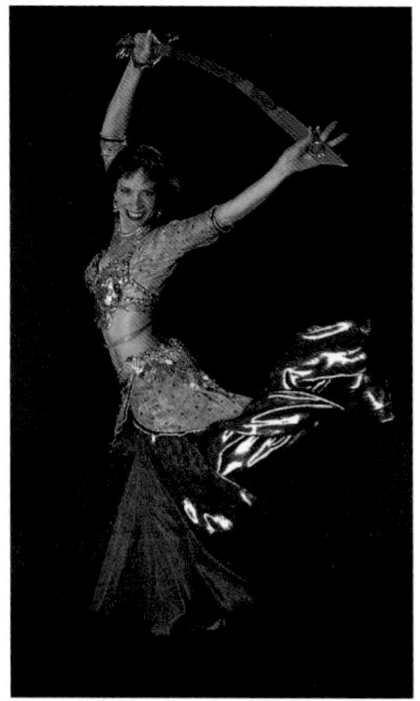

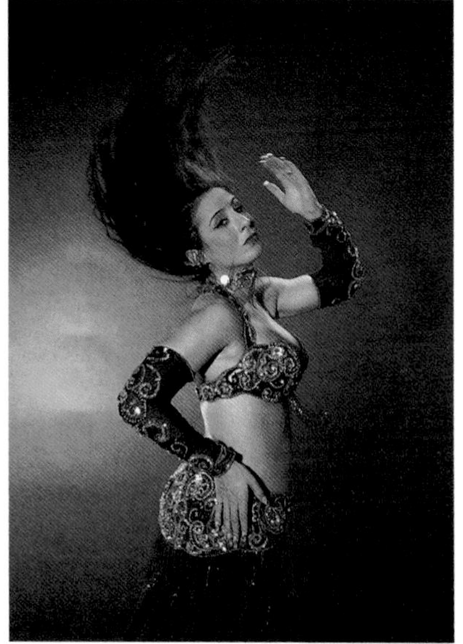

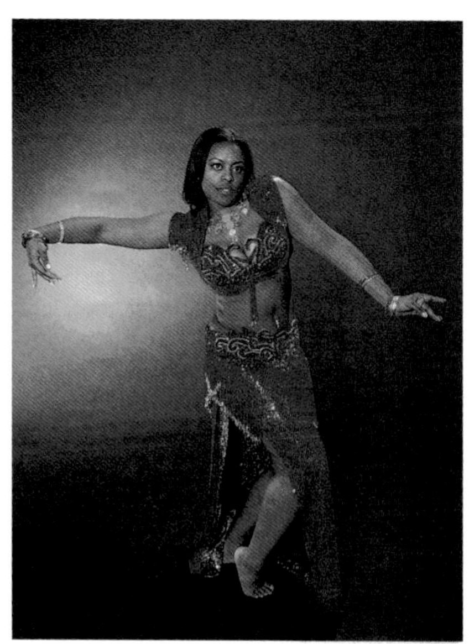

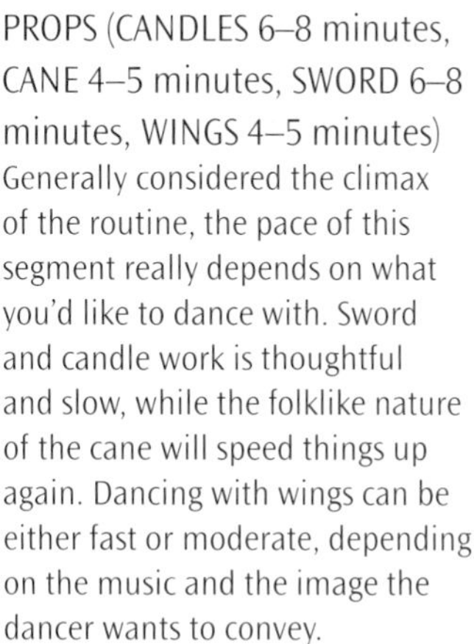

PROPS (CANDLES 6–8 minutes, CANE 4–5 minutes, SWORD 6–8 minutes, WINGS 4–5 minutes)
Generally considered the climax of the routine, the pace of this segment really depends on what you'd like to dance with. Sword and candle work is thoughtful and slow, while the folklike nature of the cane will speed things up again. Dancing with wings can be either fast or moderate, depending on the music and the image the dancer wants to convey.

FIFTH SET (2–3 minutes)
This piece is usually the moment where dancers perform what is called a drum solo. In many Middle Eastern musical compositions, there are segments when the drum beats without the accompaniment of other instruments. The rhythm becomes more lively and the dancer reflects this by changing the smoothness of her routine to sharp, passionate hip movements in time with the beat changes. The solo can also include shimmies (p.38) and anything else in the dancer's vocabulary that accents the drum set.

FINALE (2–3 minutes)
This is a farewell dance which is combined with elegant gestures of personal achievement. Common to the finale are bright smiles, winks and plenty of graceful bowing. It is also a demonstration of gratitude – to yourself and your soul for completing the routine as well as to the audience, if there is one, for watching with kindness and interest.

DANCE ROUTINES

The dance instructions on the next few pages are designed to help you practice much of what you have learned, not only to improve your skills, but also to provide you with a taste of what a routine should encompass. The dances are not subscribed any time counts so you can experiment with the speed and pauses as you wish. It's generally best for beginners to take more counts rather than less to complete a step.

Select your pieces of music: one for your entrance, one for a fast dance and another for a medium tempo veil routine. Find a long, slow composition that works well for your prop routine and a speedy number for your finale.

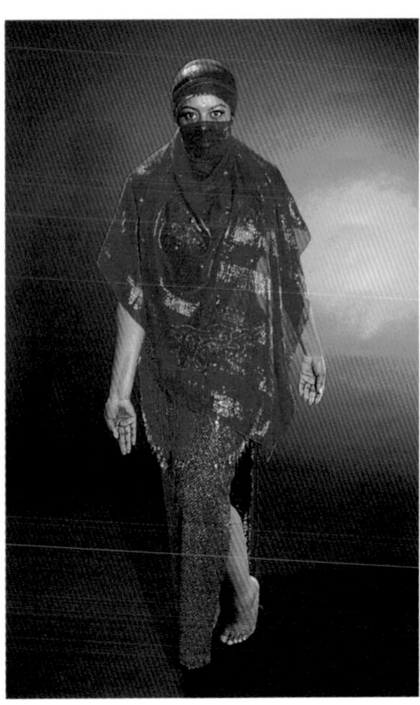

GETTING READY
Put on your veil in a style that appeals to you (pp.74–75). If you plan on dancing with zills, place them on your fingers. Select your prop and place it on the floor toward the front of your dance space – close enough to be accessible, but far enough away so you don't trip over it.

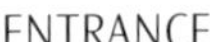

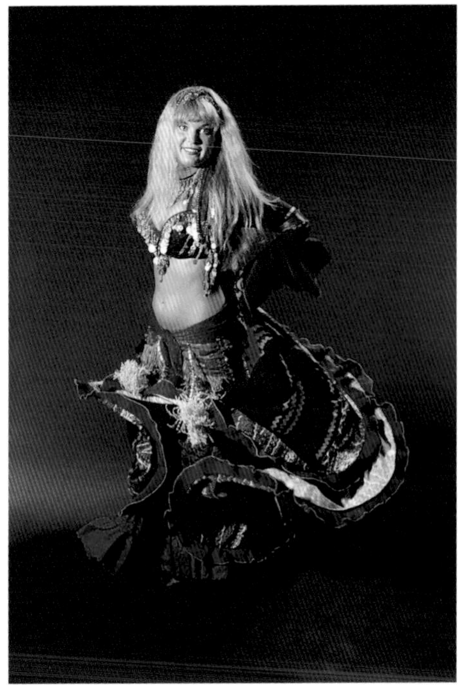

ENTRANCE
For a dramatic entrance, start your slow entrance music and get ready to become queen of the Nile! Stand outside the dance space and slowly begin a pharonic walk with prayer hands over your head. Pause and head slither left and right. When you reach the center of your space, incorporate other slow movements such as snake arms, hip rolls and undulations. Repeat your entrance until the music is finished, using the basic walk or indie cross step, along with a variety of head and arm combinations.

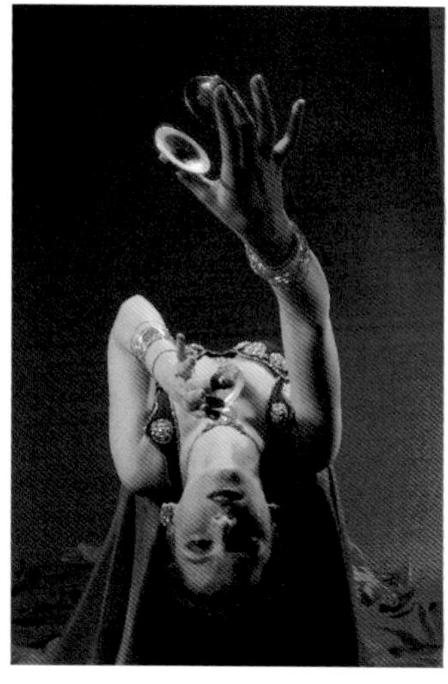

FAST DANCE WITH OR WITHOUT ZILLS

When the fast music picks up, wait until you hear the fourth solid beat before starting to dance. If playing zills, begin playing with first dance step. Then:

- 8 hip drops left
- 8 hip drops right
- 2 hip thrusts each, front, side and back on the left
- 2 hip thrusts each, front, side and back on the right
- 4 high/low hip drops left
- 4 high/low hip drops right
- Hop
- Shimmy!

- 4 kashlimar steps on the spot
- 1 box of hip snaps
- 3-point turn left
- Shoulder shake
- 3-point turn and drop right

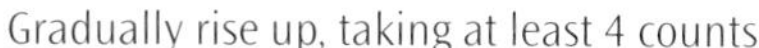

Gradually rise up, taking at least 4 counts

- 4 alternating hip rolls
- 4 hip lifts right
- 4 hip lifts left
- 2 undulations
- Hop
- Shimmy!

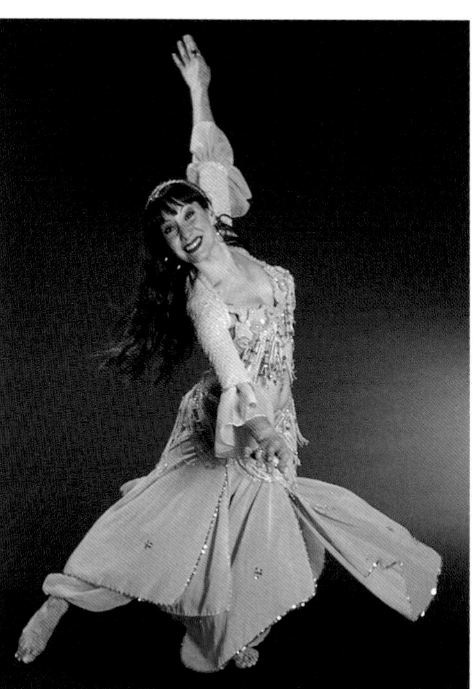

- Pivot to back
- 3 ghawazee steps back, pivot
- 3 ghawazee steps front
- 2 large hip circles
- 4 small chest circles
- 4 alternating left and right reverse hip rolls
- 2 hip twists left
- 2 hip twists right
- Hop
- Shimmy!

Repeat for practice until your music piece is complete. ▸

MEDIUM TEMPO VEIL

For the first 20 seconds of the veil music:

- 8 slow undulations, high and low, 2 each front, back, left, right
- Slow alternating snake arms front and back

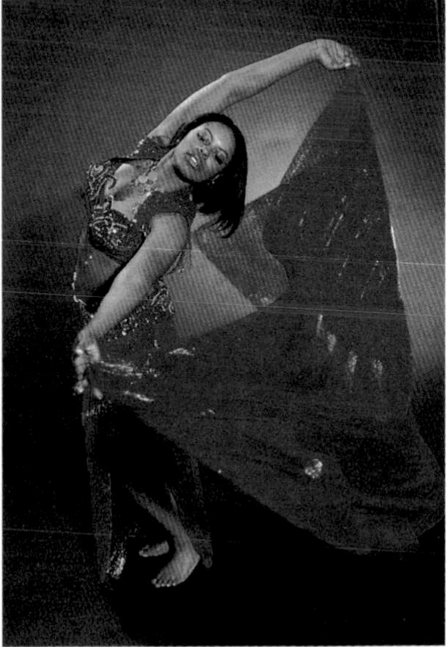

FOR THE REST OF THE MUSIC

- Unveil in steps (advance to spin when the steps are mastered)
- 1 slow veil switch left
- 2 fast veil switches right
- Cascade forward; allow veil to drop slowly
- Soft shoulder shake
- Flip into wings
- Release forward
- Cascade back
- 4 alternating left and right cascades
- Cascade forward
- Walkover
- 3 slow barrel turns left
- 3 simple turns on the spot, veil held high
- 1 body glimpse right with 2 hip drops
- 1 body glimpse left with 2 hip drops
- 1 body glimpse front with 2 undulations
- Basic walk in a wide circle with shoulder shake
- Return to center
- 3 alternating hip rolls while lowering arms to sides
- Shimmy and raise arms up slowly to center
- Spin into envelope
- 4 alternating hip rolls
- 1 box hip snaps
- Lower veil in front of eyes and peek out; wink!
- Wrap veil round head
- Shimmy and raise veil back up
- Slowly snake out of envelope
- Spin
- 2 sandstorm veils
- 1 sandstorm veil with sailing through storm
- Stop spinning abruptly and drop arms quickly to release sail
- 1 veil switch right
- 2 fast veil switches left
- Left spin through the door
- Cascade back
- 1 body glimpse front with full hip circle
- 1 body glimpse left with undulation
- 1 body glimpse right with undulation
- Wrap your arms round your chest in a hug, sway left and right leading with your shoulder

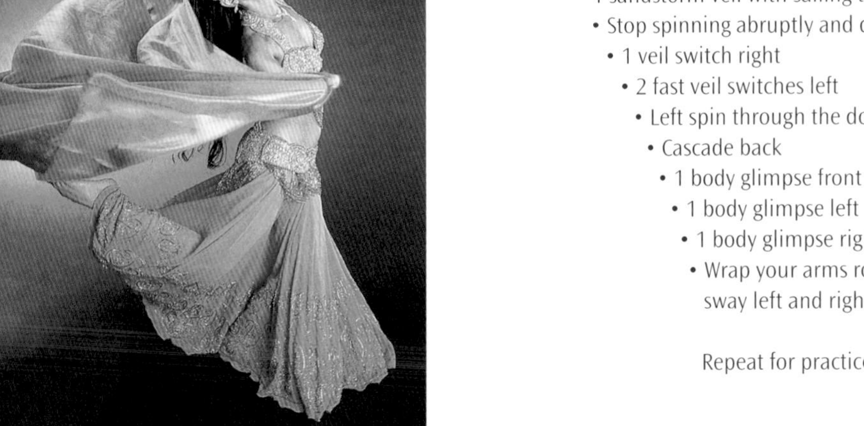

Repeat for practice until music piece is complete. ▸

VERY SLOW PROP ROUTINE

(Use with sword or candles – practice sword or unlit candles only)
Enter holding prop firmly in front of you. Take it slowly!

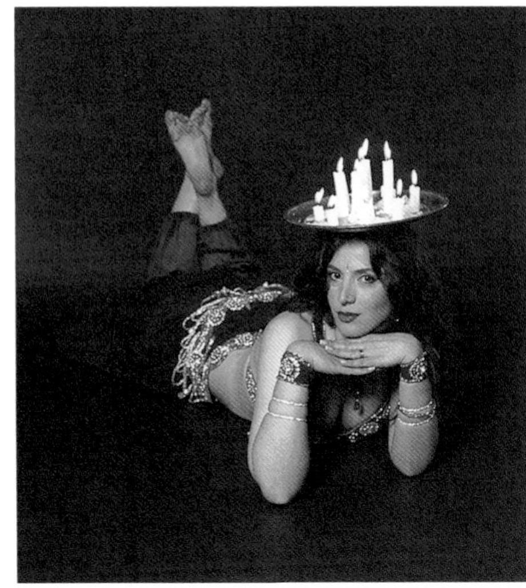

- 3 circle turns all the way around
- Hip roll in place and raise prop above your head
- 3-point turn left
- Pause
- Cobra neck slither
- 3-point turn right
- Chest circle
- Pause
- Shimmy and lower prop to waist level
- 4 alternating hip rolls
- 8 walking hip twist steps in a circle
- 4 hip drops while raising prop above head
- Half 3-point turn so your back is facing front
- Carefully place prop on head
- Very slowly complete turn
- Descend to floor
- Knee crawl
- Resurrection
- Cross kick
- Backbend undulations
- Raise to kneeling position
- Shimmy and ascend

Repeat for practice until music piece is complete.

FAST FINALE

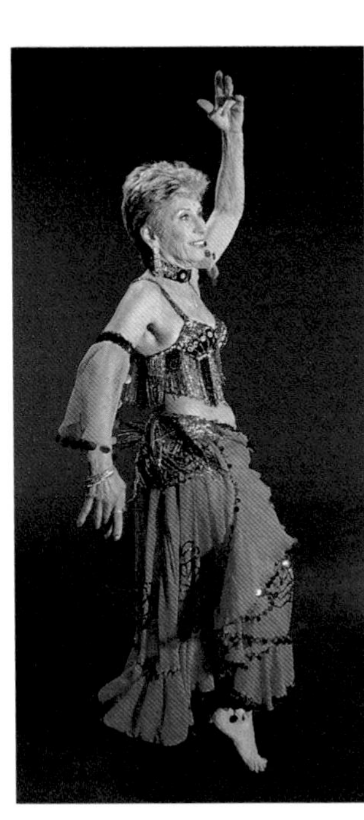

Quickly but gracefully discard your prop.
If playing zills, turn your back to the front, alternate hip rolls and return them to your fingers. Turn round and begin to play

- Ghawazee step in wide circle around dance space
- 3 alternating hip twist walks front
- Large bow
- Pivot to right
- 3 alternating hip twists right
- Shoulder shake
- Pivot to left
- 3 alternating hip twists left
- Shimmy
- Pivot to back
- 3 alternating hip twists back
- Look over shoulder to front, shoulder shake
- 3-point turn forward with drop
- Gradually come up; wink
- Large bow left
- Large bow right
- Shoulder shake, dipping left and right
- Spin
- Bow one more time and exit gracefully.

COSTUME

Costumes play a vital role in great belly dancing. They can be handmade or bought and should reflect a dancer's personal taste. There are costumes to suit all shapes and sizes. They come in every colour and in a wide range of fabrics, such as velvet, silk, chiffon and lightweight cottons. If a dancer can imagine it, it can be made! Here are a few costume types.

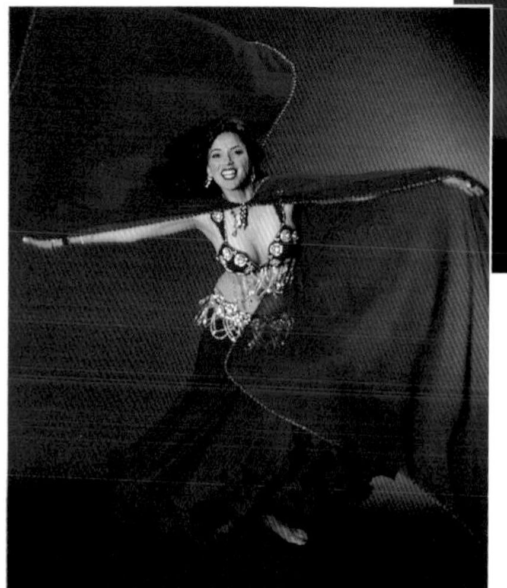

CABARET TURKISH/EGYPTIAN

These two styles are very similar. An intricately beaded and tasselled bra and belt set is draped over up to three loose skirts and/or harem pants, and worn with matching gloves, wrist cuffs, armbands and headband.

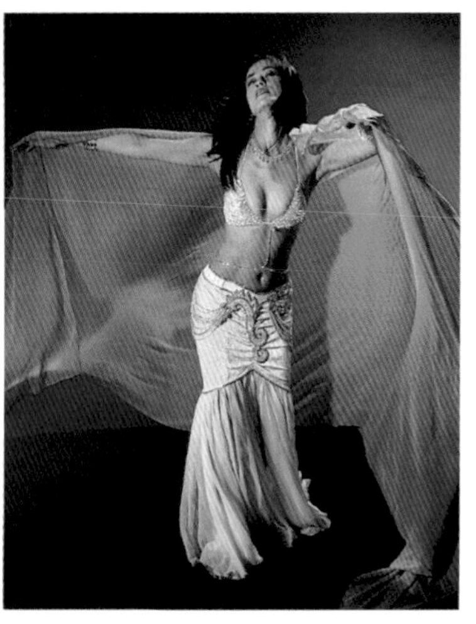

EGYPTIAN MERMAID COSTUME

Almost exactly the same as the Egyptian cabaret, the mermaid costume is distinguished by a form-fitting stretchy skirt, which smoothes over the hips and flares out at the bottom in six to eight long panels.

TRIBAL COSTUME

Lush, original adornments give tribal costumes their unique gypsy look. The top is often two pieces – a bra or choli top with a vest that closes at the solar plexus. The gored skirt is made of generous lengths of fabric so it catches the air and circles out wildly while the dancer is moving. Rich sewn-on details include coins, small bells, mirrors, cowry shells and fat dancing tassels. Some dancers also wear a decorated turban made of different scraps of brightly coloured fabrics wrapped round the head and tied at the back.

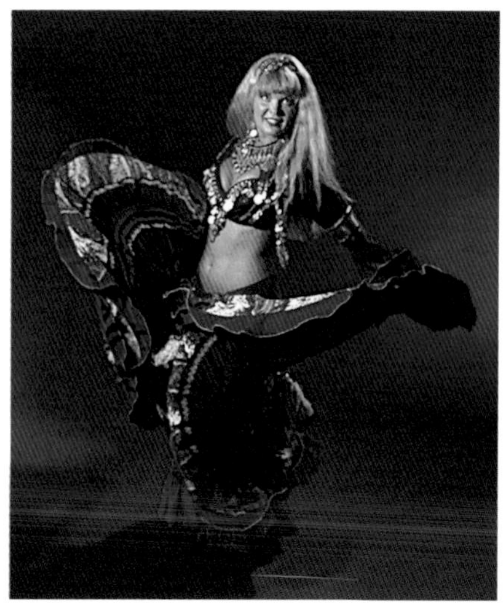

BELADI DRESS
Perfect for folk and cane dancing, the beladi dress is a classy full-length dress with long or short sleeves. A fringed, beaded or coined sash is often tied round the waist for accent.

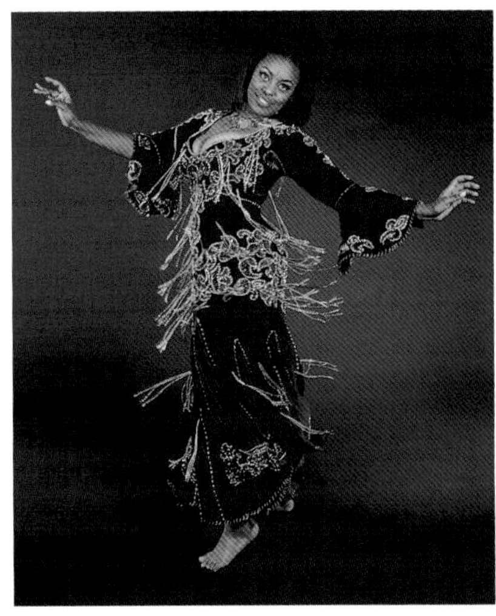

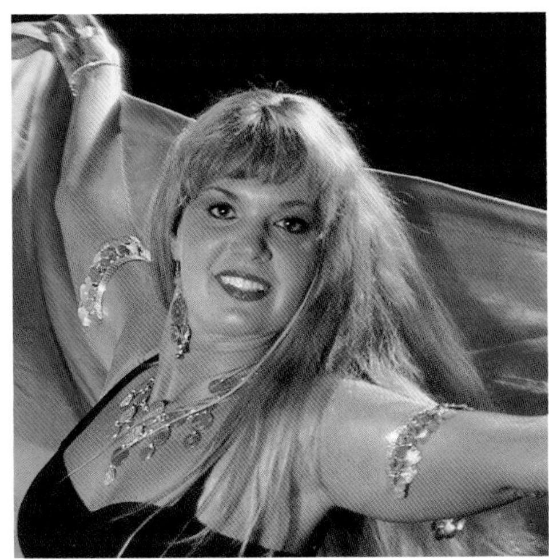

OTHER ESSENTIAL ACCESSORIES
Bracelets, necklaces, rings, earrings, armbands, anklets and a beaded headband – if the costume doesn't come with one.

OPTIONAL ACCESSORIES
Belly or toe rings.

MAKE-UP

As integral as the costume is a well made-up face. There are two main schools of thought when it comes to make-up. The first approach is simply to glamorize your current style by selecting bolder and brighter shades of cosmetics and applying them more thickly so that they show up under strong lights. Or you can play up the Oriental fantasy by applying more dramatic make-up, including heavily kohled and extended eyes, strongly arched brows and blushed cheeks. Body glitter and adhesive jewels are nice additional touches.

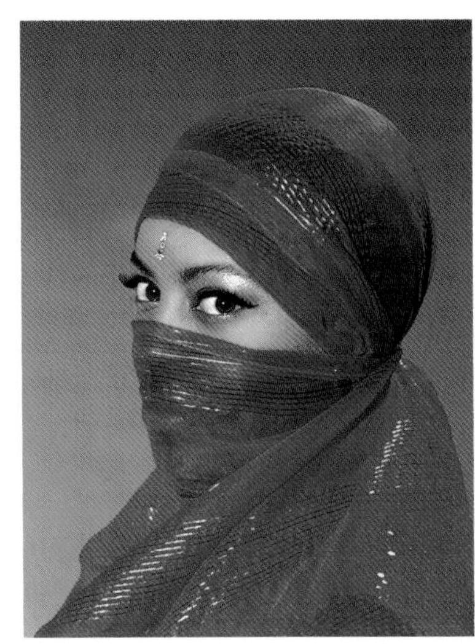

To bring out the best in every face, a dancer's make-up kit must include certain items: oil-free liquid foundation in one shade lighter than her skin colour and matching oil-free loose powder, stick and liquid eyeliner, several different shades of blusher and eye shadow, lipsticks, an eyebrow pencil that is the same shade as the darkest part of your hair, and black mascara. Waterproof cosmetics are best as they won't run when you sweat. Handy make-up accessories are eyelash curlers, cotton swabs, absorbent beauty sponges, brushes in different sizes and make-up remover for mistakes.

DANCER ETIQUETTE

At the beating heart of the dance lie its most powerful elements – mystery, fantasy and sensuality. Belly dancing is the passage to unlocking these and many other beautiful and pure emotions from within you in a unique and exclusively feminine way. Unfortunately, belly dancing suffers from an oppressive stigma, which affects its image and worldwide acceptance. To the enduring disappointment of the dancing community, many people who are unfamiliar with the history and practice of this particular style of dancing often confuse it with burlesque, striptease and other types of flesh-focused entertainment.

A combination of factors lies at the root of this debasement. Due to early European and American opposition by religious authorities and the Hollywood portrayal of belly dancers as temptresses, belly dancing became cheapened in the eyes of many as a corrupt and immoral thrill with a negative impact on society. That couldn't be further from the truth.

All forms of perfection have their cheap imitations and belly dancing is no exception. Misconduct by imposters in belly dancing costumes, as well as inappropriate portrayal of the art by the media, have diluted our legitimacy. But as long as there are still true belly dancers out there, the art of the belly dance is redeemable. The dancer herself must re-educate the viewing public and participants and show them what belly dancing really is – and what it is not.

ALWAYS BE A LADY

As a professional dancer and instructor, the single most important point that I try to impress upon my students is that first and foremost, a dancer is ALWAYS a lady. To do justice to belly dancing, her conduct must be unimpeachable under all circumstances . She must behave with elegance and dignity, and have impeccable manners. When she dances, she must be dignified, not dirty; sensuous, not sexual; and beautiful, not bawdy. There are a few etiquette techniques which if consistently followed will not only build a dancer's reputation as a legitimate artist but will also help stand as a reminder that we are not part of the sex trade world.

First, never dance for a male-only audience, such as at bachelor parties. Dancing under those circumstances creates an immediate link to the sex-for-sale concept.

Second, never allow tip money to be tucked into any part of your costume. Dancer or not, your physical being is sacred, and must not be handled by strangers in such a fashion. If you are in a public place, an appropriate alternative is to allow generous donators to sprinkle paper money down upon you in a benevolent shower. After this it is perfectly acceptable and

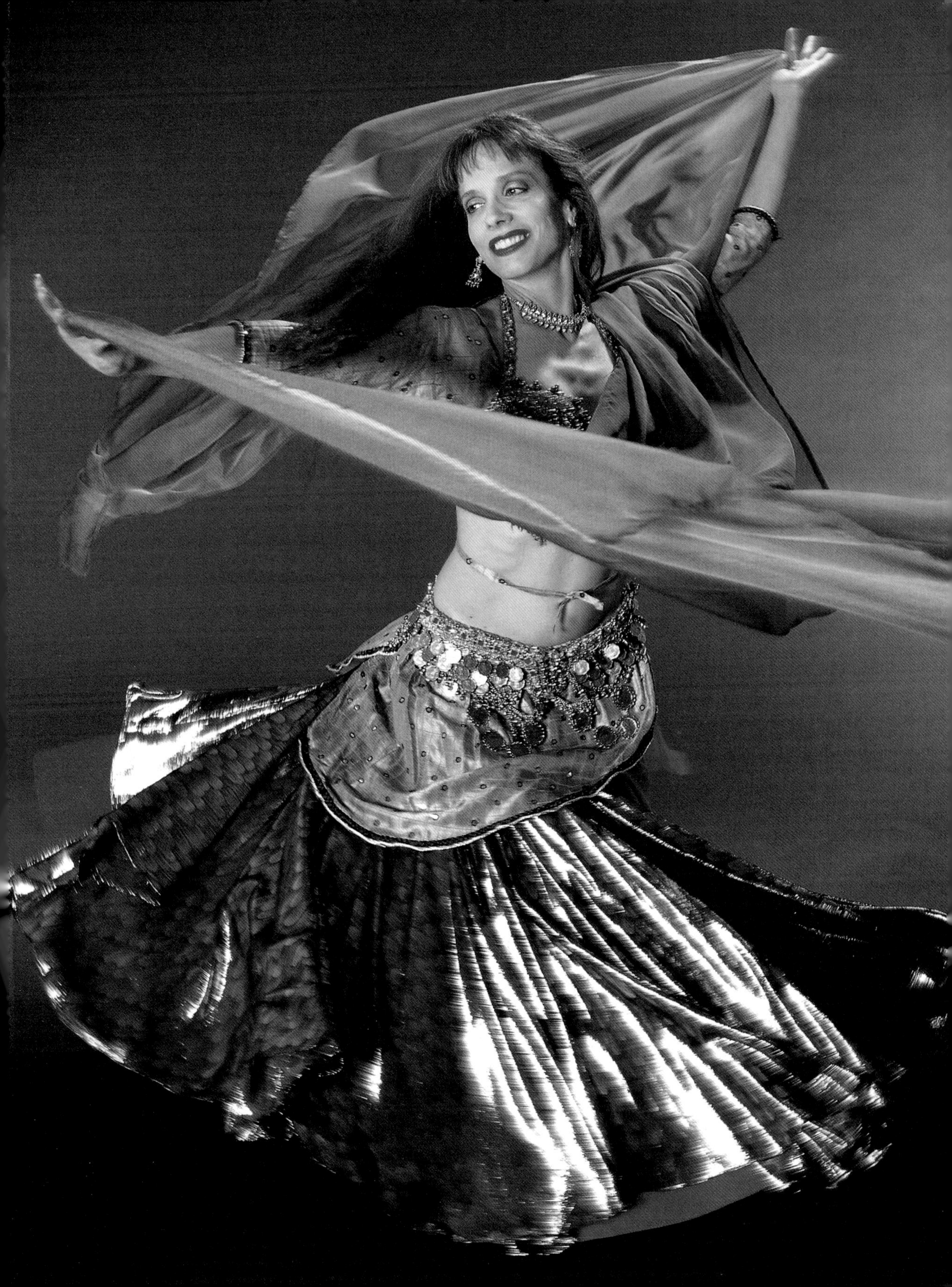

encouraged to demonstrate your gratitude with a small curtsy or graceful bow to your admirers.

Third, never stoop or kneel to gather your tips from the floor. Make a gentle request to your employer, or an employee of the establishment, to pick them up for you. If an employee collects money for you, it is courteous to give him or her a little tip in return.

Fourth, know your art inside and out from an historical perspective. Most people know nothing about belly dancing, other than what they see in the media, which is hungry for shock and scandal. Often a dancer will be faced with questions such as "Wasn't this really just a dance for harem girls to perform in front of the sultan?" or "How can you consider this to be family entertainment when your body is so exposed?" In these circumstances it is up to the dancer to remedy the misconceptions through education. Take any opportunity to explain what true belly dancing is. Know your history and be prepared to explain the facts to the curious and interested. It's a wonderful feeling when you see someone come to understand the integrity buried beneath the pop culture myth.

As you grow in the dance, keep close to your heart the awareness that the movements touch on all stages of our lifespan from birth to adolescence through to old age and passing on. Wherever you are in your own life and however you are feeling, you can pour your emotions and experience into your dancing and share them with the world. Emotions of joy, sadness and even anger can all be part of your dance.

When I stumbled into my first belly dance class I never suspected how it would enhance my life in so many positive and incredible ways. I hope with all my heart that belly dancing brings the same passion and joy to your life as it has to mine.

Resources

SUGGESTED READING

Historical

Al-Rawi, Rosina-Fawzia B., trans. by Arav, Monique, *Grandmother's Secrets: The Ancient Rituals and Healing Power of Belly Dancing*, Interlink Pub. Group, 2000

Buonaventura, Wendy and Farrah, Ibrahim, *Serpent of the Nile: Women and Dance in the Arab World*, Interlink Pub. Group, 1998

Carlton, Donna, *Looking for Little Egypt*, International Dance Discover Books, 1995

Nieuwkerk, Karin van, *"A Trade like Any Other": Female Singers and Dancers in Egypt*, Univ. of Texas Press, 1995

Richards, Tazz (editor), and Djoumahna, Kajira (introduction), *The Belly Dance Book: Rediscovering the Oldest Dance*, Backbeat Press, 2000

Stewart, Iris J., *Sacred Woman, Sacred Dance: Awakening Spirituality Through Movement & Ritual*, Inner Traditions Intl. Ltd., 2000

Thornton, Lynne, *Women As Portrayed in Orientalist Painting*, Art Books Intl. Ltd., 1996

Costuming

Brown, Barry and Brown, Dawn Devine, *Costuming from the Hip*, Ibexa Press, 1997

Brown, Barry and Brown, Dawn Devine, *From Turban to Toe Ring*, Ibexa Press, 2000

Brown, Barry and Brown, Dawn Devine, *Bedlah, Baubles, and Beads*, Ibexa Press, 2001

Personal Care

Buonaventura, Wendy and Eady, Isobel (Illustrator), *Beauty and the East: A Book of Oriental Body Care*, Interlink Pub. Group, 2000

MAGAZINES

Bennu
Associated Artists of Middle Eastern Dance Inc.
A non-profit organization
72 Park Terrace West, Suite E48
New York, NY 10034-1351

Habibi
PO Box 42018
Eugene, OR 97404

Zaghareet!
P.O. Box 1809
Elizabeth City, NC 27906

SHOPPING ABROAD

Egypt
Mr Mahmoud Abd El Ghaffar
"Al-Wikalah"
75 Gawfar El Qayid St
Al-Musky
Al-Azhar
Cairo, Egypt
Tel: 20 2 589 7443
Fax: 20 2 390 0357

Turkey
Madame Bella
"Boutique Bella"
Fulya Cad. Erse Han No. 3-5 D.16
Mecidiyeköy, Istanbul
Turkey
Tel: 90 212 272 2029,
Fax: 90 212 288-3699

COSTUMES
Costumes online USA
Ready-made designs
www.topkapidesigns.com (Turkish)
www.home.earthlink.net (Turkish)
www.egyptworld.com (Egyptian)
www.pyramidimports.com (Egyptian)

Nourhan Sharif Dancewear
http://www.nourhansharif.com

Alia Michelle Designs
http://aliamdesigns.com/

Custom-made designs
http://www.aliamdesigns.com/
www.domba.com

Costumes online UK
www.whirling-dervish.co.uk
www.khalganikostumes.com
www.theshimmyshop.co.uk
www.faridadance.com

CLASSES
Try looking at the links listed below or get in touch with your local leisure center or dance school for classes

Information online USA
www.bellydanceny.com

Information online UK
www.mosaicdance.org
www.footwork.org/ghazala/main.htm
http://www.shira.net/dir-uk.htm (directory of instructors)
Council for dance education and training
http://www.cdet.org.uk/index2.htm

BELLY DANCERS
www.dancingmoonlight.com (author's website)
www.geocities.com/mimibellydance
www.enchantressofbioluminosity.com/
www.rajadance.com
www.bellydancersonline.com
http://www.bellydancer.info/
www.vers.com/kanari
www.mysticbellydancer.com

MUSIC
Omar Faruk Tekbilek (Turkish)
Faruk has 10 fabulous CDs. His soulful voice and compositions never fail to inspire.
My personal favourites are
Dance into Eternity
Cresent Moon
Alif
www.omarfaruktekbilek.com

Hossam Ramzy (Egyptian)
Hossam is world famous for his music. His perfect percussion rhythms are wonderful to learn from. My personal favourites are:
Secrets of the Eye
Source of Fire
Rhythms of the Nile

Jehan Kemal (fusion)
Not only an utterly stunning dancer, Jehan has a mysterious and spiritual voice that is the very epitome of femininity in the dance.
My personal favourites are:
The Goddess Dance series
Sacred Waters
Heartbeat
www.jehanarts.com

Index

AUTHOR'S ACKNOWLEDGMENTS

My endless love and gratitude first and foremost to my husband, whose unwavering support and dedication I cannot not live without.

Deep and warm appreciation to my cakes at Gaia Books, Sara and Jinny, who held my hand through this whole project even though they are on the other side of the Atlantic.

Many loving thanks to my family, immediate and extended, who always believe I can do anything. And tender gratefulness to my dear Kindred Spirits, especially The Neon, whose companionship are ever my safe havens.

PUBLISHER'S ACKNOWLEDGMENTS

Gaia Books would like to thank the following for their help in the making of this book: Naia, Mimi, Andrea Anwar, Raja, Leyla, Kanari, Fahdida, Elisabeth, Aquila and Heidi, who modelled and danced for the step by step photographs; Heidi Steinberg and Joey McGill for make-up; Nourhan Sharif Dancewear and Alia Michelle Designs for costumes; Claire Hayward and Ann Marie Philip for design assistance; Joel Porter for technical support; Elizabeth Wiggans for compiling the index; Michael Beacom and Jeff Solomon at Sterling.

Photographic credits: All photographs are by Sarah Skinner except for those on pages 9, 10 and 11 from the Mary Evans Picture Library. Sarah Skinner would like to give special thanks to Kevin Fox, Ursula Jones and Jack Skinner.